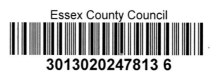

THE DEVIL'S DOCTORS

*For Fang Fang
and William*

THE DEVIL'S DOCTORS

Japanese Human Experiments on Allied Prisoners of War

Mark Felton

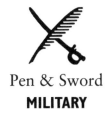

Pen & Sword
MILITARY

First published in Great Britain in 2012 by
Pen & Sword Military
an imprint of
Pen & Sword Books Ltd
47 Church Street
Barnsley
South Yorkshire
S70 2AS

Copyright © Mark Felton, 2012

ISBN: 978-1-84884-479-7

The right of Mark Felton to be identified as Author of this Work has been asserted by him in accordance with the Copyright, Designs and Patents Act 1988.

A CIP catalogue record for this book is
available from the British Library.

All rights reserved. No part of this book may be reproduced or transmitted in any form or by any means, electronic or mechanical including photocopying, recording or by any information storage and retrieval system, without permission from the Publisher in writing.

Typeset in 11/13pt Palatino by
Concept, Huddersfield, West Yorkshire

Printed and bound in England by
CPI Group (UK) Ltd, Croydon, CR0 4YY

Pen & Sword Books Ltd incorporates the Imprints of Pen & Sword Aviation, Pen & Sword Family History, Pen & Sword Maritime, Pen & Sword Military, Pen & Sword Discovery, Wharncliffe Local History, Wharncliffe True Crime, Wharncliffe Transport, Pen & Sword Select, Pen & Sword Military Classics, Leo Cooper, The Praetorian Press, Remember When, Seaforth Publishing and Frontline Publishing.

For a complete list of Pen & Sword titles please contact
PEN & SWORD BOOKS LIMITED
47 Church Street, Barnsley, South Yorkshire, S70 2AS, England
E-mail: enquiries@pen-and-sword.co.uk
Website: www.pen-and-sword.co.uk

Contents

Acknowledgements		vi
Introduction		1
1	The Seeds of Death	9
2	Paris of the Orient	21
3	Blood Harvest	31
4	The Camp	40
5	Forced Labour	62
6	Guinea Pigs	74
7	Precedents and Paper Trails	100
8	Flamingo	113
9	Reaping the Whirlwind	122
10	Operation 'PX'	144
11	Dark Harvest	158
Conclusion		165
Appendix A		171
Appendix B		173
Appendix C		177
Appendix D		179
Notes		184
Index		194

Acknowledgements

I should like to express my gratitude to the following individuals, institutions and organisations who have given so freely of their time in answering my questions and aiding my research for this book. Many thanks to Lieutenant-Colonel Jonathan Knowles of the Royal Army Ordnance Corps Association; Justin Saddington of the National Army Museum; Michael Hurst, MBE, the Director of the Taiwan POW Camps Memorial Society; Rod Suddaby and Simon Offord at the Imperial War Museum in London. My particular thanks go to Pat Wang and the Mukden Prisoner of War Remembrance Society which has managed to preserve the remnants of the Mukden Camp as an excellent and informative museum with the assistance of the Chinese authorities in Shenyang. Shelly and Sue Zimbler of the Mukden Survivors' & Descendants Group have been wonderful, and I should like to thank them very much. The assistance of Ron Taylor and the Far East Prisoners of War Association has been, as usual, invaluable during the course of researching this book, and both you and your organisation have my warmest gratitude. Many thanks also to Maurice Christie, author of *Operation Scapula*. My wife Fang Fang has acted as a brilliant research assistant and translator during the course of this project, enabling the Chinese side of the Unit 731 debate to be more fully explored, and Chinese academics and writers consulted. She did all of this in the midst of her busy career as well as finding the time to listen to my many ideas and theories, and has helped me to stay focused during the gestation of this book. Many thanks to Shirley Felton who has acted as an unpaid research assistant in Britain and tracked down innumerable published

Acknowledgements

sources and very kindly sent so much material to me in Shanghai. Finally, my warmest thanks to Brigadier Henry Wilson, Matt Jones for all their hard work on this project and the excellent team at Pen & Sword Books, and my editor Sue Blackhall.

Introduction

We removed some of the organs and amputated legs and arms. Two of the victims were young women, 18 or 19 years old. I hesitate to say it but we opened up their wombs to show the younger soldiers. They knew little about women – it was sex education.

Unit 731 veteran Akira Makino, March 2007

With their breath streaming like smoke into the freezing air, a small group of American prisoners bundled up in winter coats and caps, stacked the bodies of their comrades like cordwood in a long wooden hut. The bodies had been wrapped in dirty sheets and taken directly from the camp's rudimentary hospital to the storeroom. There they would reside for the remainder of the harsh Manchurian winter and be denied a Christian burial on the orders of the Japanese camp commandant. Something unseen was stalking the prisoners at Mukden Camp, a collection of dilapidated Chinese barracks that had been turned into a temporary prisoner-of-war camp by the Japanese in 1942; an as yet unidentified disease that was carrying off American inmates with horrific regularity. Each day the senior British officer in the camp, Major Robert Peaty, concealed himself quietly inside his bunk and carefully recorded the numbers of deceased, normally between one and three young men a day. The men had all developed severe diarrhoea, had sickened and died quickly. Peaty had also noted the strange visits to the camp by teams of Japanese doctors, and the barrage of hypodermic injections all the nationalities inside the camp had received.

The Devil's Doctors

Come the spring, and the same team of American prisoners who had gently placed their dead comrades bodies into winter storage on the orders of the Japanese, were now told to bring the defrosted cadavers out of the hut and place them carefully on to a table that had been set up under the crisp spring sunshine. The naked bodies were unwrapped and carefully examined by murmuring Japanese Army surgeons. Without preamble, incisions were made, organs removed and samples carefully marked, as the Allied prisoners stood silently watching this final desecration of their dead. Once the autopsies were complete, the bodies were finally released for burial and the Japanese medical personnel left the camp with their grim specimens carefully logged in glass jars and phials. But the deaths inside the camp continued, and whatever was killing the Allied prisoners at the Mukden Camp continued its microbial work in silence as Major Peaty continued to note in pencil each daily fatality in his secret diary.

In China today there is a place that is so loathed and hated. Located in the northern city of Pingfan near Harbin in Heilongjiang Province, a place that has come to sum up for many Chinese the true face of the Japanese aggression that was unleashed against the nation seventy years ago. It ranks alongside the massacre memorial hall located in the busy city of Nanjing as representative of all the sufferings heaped upon the Chinese people by Imperial Japan between 1931 and 1945. It also remains as one of the great stumbling blocks between China and Japan ever reaching a true *entente* in the twenty-first century. It is a collection of sturdy redbrick buildings that carries the most infamous three-number identifier in history – Unit 731.

The buildings at Pingfan are the remains of a gigantic experiment in biological and chemical warfare conducted by the Japanese military in occupied Manchuria. Many thousands of innocent people, from babies and young children, to adults of several nations, a list that has consistently included rumours of Allied prisoners-of-war, were put to death at the Pingfan facility in the name of science. Japanese military doctors, with the assistance of the *Kempeitai* military police, were permitted to conduct every sort of medical experiment on live human beings; experiments that are normally proscribed by law, morality and political and public revulsion. They were as free to play with lives in order to further scientific understanding as the most notorious of the SS

Introduction

doctors in the Nazi concentration camps, to push the boundaries of our understanding of human beings, and of human resistance to disease, infection and extremes of temperature, altitude and privation.

At Pingfan, secrets were layered upon secrets until myths were created that endure to the present day. We know that thousands of Chinese citizens perished in the most horrid manner in this factory of death. We know that White Russian and later Soviet citizens also disappeared into its operating rooms and onto its test ranges. And we have some tantalizing clues that hint that perhaps American and British prisoners-of-war also died inside its compounds and bunkers.

The experience of Allied POWs in Japanese hands has gone down in history as a very dark period, marked by a rejection of the agreed practices for the treatment of enemy captives and civilians. The disclosure that British and American soldiers also perished in a human medical-experimentation programme, and that those responsible were never properly punished, would have to be one of the last terrible secrets of the Second World War. This book attempts to disentangle fact from the many fictions that have grown up around this emotive subject, and to come to some reasonable conclusions about what did actually happen. The results of this process suggest that the more outlandish fictions were not so far from the mark as previously thought.

The Japanese desperately tried to cover the crimes of Unit 731 when the war came to a bloody end with the twin holocausts of Hiroshima and Nagasaki in August 1945, but much of their facility, too well-built to be easily demolished, survived to stand testimony into the twenty-first century to Japan's engineered holocaust upon the innocent. So powerful is Unit 731's historical legacy that the events at Pingfan and a host of other locations under its authority, continue to sour Sino-Japanese relations in the present day. The Japanese officially deny much of what happened at Pingfan and elsewhere, while the Chinese government, for its own self-serving reasons, is determined that its people should never forget what happened. The American and British governments officially have no interest in the matter, preferring to deny the strong evidence that shows a direct link between Unit 731 and Allied prisoners-of-war. They have chosen to not establish that link formally, and to create further confusion with much of the pertinent documentation that could very well contain direct evidence of such a link still either classified or missing.

This book focuses much of its attention on one particular POW camp, and what occurred inside this camp provides some of the most compelling evidence for Allied POWs having been unknowingly inducted into Unit 731's research programme. In the wooden hutted Mukden Camp in the far north of China, several thousand Allied POWs lived in harsh and difficult conditions between 1942 and their liberation in late August 1945. During the winter they froze and during the summer they baked, the region's weather systems just one more threat to their lives since their capture by the Japanese during the great Allied defeats in Asia in 1941–42. Nearly every day the prisoners rose early and filed off to labour in a series of privately-owned Japanese factories, yet another violation of agreements that determined the treatment of enemy combatants. They were not particularly well fed, and sometimes their guards would beat or humiliate them. You have probably read something like this before, and certainly if you have ever read a book or seen a film that discusses the treatment of prisoners by the Japanese.

The Mukden Camp lay in that part of Asia that used to be called Manchuria before the war, and is today three separate but related provinces, Liaoning, Heilongjiang and Jilin, located in the high north of the People's Republic of China that border Mongolia and Russia. It was from this area that the last Imperial dynasty of China, the Manchus, swept south and conquered the Celestial Empire in the seventeenth century, and whose last representative, the boy emperor Pu Yi, was swept aside by the new republic in 1912. The camp buildings, camp routine, camp diet and camp brutality were neither particularly worse than any other Japanese POW camp of the period, and neither were they unique in any respect save for one. The camp, named after the nearest Manchurian city, Mukden (renamed Shenyang by the Communists in 1949), has become a rather enigmatic place for historians; a place where medical experiments may have been performed, and where the Japanese may have extended Unit 731's research to include Caucasian soldiers.

For over sixty years rumours have persisted that the Japanese experimented on Allied POWs, and the name that has consistently been linked with the Mukden Camp and its tragic inhabitants is

Introduction

'Unit 731', itself still a largely enigmatic and mysterious organisation. Responsible for some of the very worst outrages against morality ever conceived, what was done at Unit 731 was nothing less than a horrific amalgam of sadism, murder and science gone very, very wrong. The suggestion that the malignant tendrils of this most reviled organisation had wrapped themselves around an Allied POW camp are almost fantastical to contemplate – but, as this book will demonstrate – not completely beyond the realms of chilling reality. As mentioned above, the subject remains a sensitive one and you will find no official admissions by the American or British governments of Unit 731's use of Allied POWs in its bizarre research programme. But so many documents remain classified, so many questions remain resolutely unanswered, and so many tantalizing clues remain scattered throughout witness statements, diaries, documents and books that it is also not beyond the realm of fantasy to suggest that something was indeed very different in the Mukden Camp. Perhaps the Mukden Camp was that link between young men from the United States, Britain, Australia, New Zealand and Holland, and some of the most evil perpetrators of pseudo-science who have ever walked the earth.

This book has a simple, but hopefully intriguing and thought-provoking, premise. It is historical fact that in 1942, during the darkest days of the Second World War in Asia following catastrophic Allied defeats, a group of American, British, and Australian prisoners-of-war, along with a smattering of New Zealanders and Dutch, were brought from two very different tropical locations to the Mukden Camp in the high north of China. There were no other Allied POW centres that were located nearby and, indeed, the camp was hundreds of miles from the closest concentration of Caucasian prisoners at Woosung, outside Shanghai in central China. The Japanese mystifyingly went to an awful lot of trouble and expense to move just a few thousand Allied soldiers to Mukden, a journey that involved ships and trains, and visits to Singapore, the Philippines, Japan, Korea and finally Manchuria. During the journey the prison ship risked being sunk by Allied submarines, and the Japanese risked losing more of their human cargo to disease.

This book states a bold premise that explains why the Japanese went to so much expense and effort to move a few thousand

Allied POWs to Manchuria. It was so they might provide the human test subjects for a series of life-threatening biological warfare tests that were conducted by the shadowy and nefarious Unit 731. Mukden Camp was a few hundred miles south of Unit 731's main research centre at Pingfan, but right next door to another of its outstations, the Mukden Military Hospital.

The Japanese required Caucasian test subjects so that they could further their understanding of the effectiveness of potential biological weapons they were busy developing for battlefield use against their many enemies. The Japanese, since the early 1930s, had been illegally experimenting with deadly bacilli in an effort to create devastating weapons. Under the leadership of a brilliant but morally bankrupt scientist, Dr. Shiro Ishii, Unit 731 had used human experimentation as the standard means of discovering how diseases destroyed the human body. Thousands of men, women and children had been sacrificed to these secret and diabolical experiments. The Japanese had managed to develop many of the weapons they desired from these tests, and then used them on local villages and towns in China with extremely lethal effect. Hundreds of thousands of Chinese had been deliberately murdered by diseases which had been cynically introduced to the local environment by Unit 731 scientists, either through aerial sprays and special ceramic bombs, or through poisoning water sources and food. The success of this programme had shown the Japanese High Command the extreme value of biological warfare weapons. By 1944, when Japan was losing the war against the United States and the British Commonwealth, its leaders, like their Nazi allies, increasingly turned to 'wonder weapons' in the hope of reversing the inevitable defeat. Working in close technical and scientific cooperation with Germany, jet fighters and early cruise missiles were developed, as well as advanced submarines and biological warfare (BW) weapons. As the war progressed, the Japanese High Command began to seriously consider using BW weapons against the United States, and, as we shall see, they managed to develop novel ways to make this goal a horrific reality. It is no coincidence that many of the American veterans who were held prisoner at Mukden have recounted how medical tests reached a peak in 1943 – at exactly the same time Japan was developing the means to deliver deadly BW weapons to the American home front.

Introduction

The available evidence from American, British and Japanese sources suggests that the Japanese wanted to test how Caucasians stood up to the same diseases which they had been testing up to that point on mostly Asian prisoners in Manchuria. It would have appeared a logical and sensible move if a BW campaign was being formulated against targets in the United States, not to mention their possible use on the battlefields of the Pacific and Burma.

Historians admit that although *prima facie* evidence for Japanese experiments on Allied POWs is persuasive and intriguing, there is little direct evidence that has survived that definitively answers the question of whether Unit 731 conducted tests on American and British POWs at the Mukden Camp. But there is incontrovertible evidence that Japanese physicians conducted tests on American, British and Australian POWs in other parts of Asia, thereby setting a precedent. There is oral testimony from Japanese who worked at Unit 731 which states unequivocally that scientists performed tests on Allied POWs at Mukden. There are a whole series of unusual medical occurrences at the Mukden Camp which certainly make it unique in the history of Japanese POW camps, occurrences that point to it being an organised experimentation programme being undertaken by an outside party. In fact, we might state with some authority, and this will certainly become evident as the story of what occurred inside the Mukden Camp unfolds across the following chapters, that the camp was a very strange place indeed.

The evidence has been scattered across half a world since the end of the war, and has never before been completely reassembled to present a compelling insight into the Japanese BW programme and its relationship with the poor souls imprisoned inside the Mukden Camp. The most compelling part of the story is how each disparate strand of evidence, both oral and written, from many different nationalities and times, crucially corroborates each other, providing us with a good chance of solving once and for all the intriguing historical question of whether Allied POWs were also victims of Unit 731, alongside the many Asians who perished in its hands.

There is well-documented evidence that the Japanese High Command seriously considered ordering the deployment of BW weapons against the mainland of the United States in the latter part of the war, and that they ordered a massive diversion of manpower, money and resources to the construction of munitions delivery systems to make such a plan a reality. And there is strong evidence of a wide-ranging cover-up of Japan's wartime human experimentation programme by the United States and British governments in the immediate postwar period, when, through backstairs deals, the Allies granted Dr. Ishii and his team of murderers blanket immunity from prosecution in return for all of their secret data derived from so much suffering and cruelty. This cover-up continues even six decades after the end of the war with many documents still classified or missing completely from files on the subject, posing the obvious question about what are the American and British governments concealing.

The overwhelming thread to this story is one of logic. Military's seldom create expensive research programmes on a whim, and the available evidence strongly suggests that Allied POWs were the victims of Unit 731's BW warfare programme. The coincidences are just too many, and the inconsistencies inherent in the arguments that have been put forward by those who deny the experiments are also too many. It was perhaps the darkest part of the hellish story of Allied POWs in the hands of the Japanese, and perhaps it remains the most enigmatic story – but taken together for the first time, the truth is disturbingly and coldly *logical*.

Chapter 1

The Seeds of Death

Biological warfare must possess distinct possibilities otherwise it would not have been outlawed by the League of Nations.

Captain Shiro Ishii, 1931

The big transport ship lurched through the heavy waves, its engines noisily turning the screws that churned the water at the stern into angry white foam. The ship was filthy and dilapidated, its sides streaked with rust, and its superstructure grimy and encrusted with salt spray. Above the superstructure a single smokestack coughed thick, black smoke into the sky as the ship pounded relentlessly north. Down in the ship's holds was a scene reminiscent of the Middle Passage – hundreds upon hundreds of white men crammed so tightly into the filthy and dark holds that they could barely find space to lie down on the hard metal deck plates. Accompanying the vision of overcrowding was a riotous cacophony of noises – moaning, coughing, shouting, murmuring and sometimes retching. The smell was rank, an accumulation of unwashed bodies, human excrement and vomit.

Peering down from the open hatches above were the laughing faces of Japanese soldiers, who smoked and chatted high above their prisoners. The 'slaves' whose grimy, white faces occasionally stared up at the guards with undisguised fear and loathing, were American soldiers, captured at the conclusion of the fight for the Philippines; the ragged survivors of an army that had been humbled in battle against a foe most had hitherto thought its inferior in every way, and then brutalized in captivity by an enemy many now thought beyond the pale of humanity. These prisoners were destined for a new camp and a new purpose in the Japanese war plan. For many of them, this journey to the north was to be their last. It was a one-way ticket to hell.

As with many things in early twentieth-century Japan, an interest in chemical and biological warfare came about through fear. The fear was that the Western Powers, particularly Britain and the United States – who dominated Asia at the time and who had developed these fearsome weapons first and also used them effectively during the First World War – would advance far ahead of the Japanese in this technology. The Japanese chemical and biological warfare programme was the brainchild of one rather eccentric doctor who made it his life's work to create weapons of such destructive capacity that his name and the institution that he founded would live on in infamy. His name was Dr. Shiro Ishii, and the organisation he created would come to be known to the world as Unit 731.

When Japanese diplomats had signed the Geneva Convention in 1925, they had signed away their legal right to develop or deploy chemical and biological weapons, along with all of the other countries that had put ink to paper. Thirty-five-year-old microbiologist Ishii, who had just graduated from the prestigious Kyushu Imperial University and joined the army as a medical officer, had what can only be described as a kind of 'eureka' moment when he read a report about the Convention and the weapons that it prohibited, penned by a young Japanese army officer named Lieutenant Harada, who had accompanied the diplomats as an attaché to Switzerland in 1925. The brilliant, though highly unorthodox, Ishii, who wore round wire-framed glasses and had thick, black hair, could see that chemical, and especially biological warfare (BW), weapons were immensely powerful tools of war. The framers of the Geneva Convention were influenced in their decision to ban such weapons, and research into them, by the experiences of the First World War when Mustard Gas had been widely used. They also feared a return of the Black Death, as nations with BW weapons had the potential to kill millions with the bubonic plague and other hideous forms of weaponized bacilli. The fear was similar to that expressed over the supposed 'Weapons of Mass Destruction' that led to war in Iraq in 2003 when the United States and Britain became convinced that Saddam Hussein possessed a formidable arsenal of these Domesday weapons. The nations of the world in 1925 considered such weapons to be immoral and unnecessary. The fact that they had been specifically banned spoke directly to Ishii's perverted thought process. They had been outlawed specifically because they were so powerful – and logically it made perfect sense that Japan should have them.

Ishii, a fervent nationalist who believed that Japan had the right to build an empire in Asia, led a one-man crusade for several years, badgering and pestering generals and colonels for interviews where he quickly and eloquently laid out his ideas for developing BW weapons in secret. It would give Japan the military edge over its likely future enemies, not least among them the Western Powers and the dreaded Soviet Union. And Ishii argued vehemently that Japan was well within her rights to develop BW weapons because the Western Powers were basically operating a hypocritical policy. He could point to the true fact that countries like Britain and Germany had signed the 1899 Hague Convention that had specifically banned chemical weapons research, but then deployed such weapons on the Western Front during the Great War. Who was to say whether these nations, and others, were not already secretly doing the same again following the Geneva Convention? High-blown diplomatic rhetoric could have masked more sinister programmes by Japan's competitors. Ishii had a point; for although BW research was expressly forbidden, the British certainly maintained a skeleton programme at their main research facility at Porton Down in Wiltshire between the wars, allowing for its full reactivation as soon as Germany invaded Poland in 1939. The Americans, too, were as equally covert with their programmes.

Unfortunately for Shiro Ishii, the timing of his presentations and arguments to the Japanese high command was not quite right. The military had yet to move to the absolute centre of Japanese politics where it could dictate the nation's destiny, and the democratically elected government was relatively peaceful and law-abiding on the international stage, apart from some occasional nationalistic forays into Korea and Manchuria during the 1920s.

One definite advantage Ishii identified was that Japan in the 1920s was one of the world's leaders in medical and drug technologies, providing plenty of potential researchers and research centres should his plans have come to fruition. The Japanese were also especially proud of their humane treatment of German and Austro-Hungarian POWs that had been captured in China during the Great War. The behaviour of the Japanese had been beyond reproach, and a very far cry from how the nation would treat its captured enemies over the coming two decades. Among the international community of nations, Japan stood high both morally and scientifically. This would change quite dramatically over the coming ten years.

Was Shiro Ishii's plan to develop chemical and BW weapons completely reprehensible, and was he 'evil' in the classic sense of the word? What happened later at Unit 731 and at other attached units across Asia certainly suggests that Ishii and his comrades cared little about the individual lives of those they experimented on. But some of Ishii's psychology can be explained. Born into a noble *samurai* family just outside of Tokyo in 1892, Ishii hailed from the warrior class which had ruled Japan for centuries with the total obedience of the Japanese people. The Meiji Restoration in 1868 that had ushered in a newly-industrialized and progressively more democratic Japan, replaced a hereditary military dictator called the *Shogun* with a revitalized constitutional monarchy in the form of a compliant Emperor. But the Meiji Restoration had actually changed very little in the way of attitudes, and instead, created a new powerful elite that ran the government and the economy. It was progressive anti-*Shogun samurai* families who had benefitted from the opening up of Japan to Western ideas and technology, and it was these progressives who had formed the first governments, and the first major companies – a very good example being Mitsubishi, the company that was later accused of having exploited American, British and Australian prisoners-of-war as forced labourers at Mukden. The *samurai* formed the officer corps of the army and the navy, and they still enjoyed a pre-eminent status, just as the sons of aristocrats and the landed gentry continued to dominate the top universities, the officer corps and the government of Great Britain, the world's foremost industrialized nation at the time. Ishii had been raised with servants looking after his daily needs, and he had been educated to be aware and proud of his social position. 'Such rules against fraternizing with the so-called lower classes ... must have made a deep impression on Ishii,' writes Daniel Barenblatt in his seminal book *A Plague upon Humanity*. 'It made it all the easier for him and the other Japanese perpetrators of lethal human experimentation to descend into a callous disregard for human life.'[1] Of course, merely being born into a gentrified family does not mean that one inherits a psychopathic or sociopathic mentality. Ishii was heavily influenced by his own personal ambitions and ultra-nationalism, and by the fact that later in his career, superior officers encouraging his experiments in order that Japan would win the war, surrounded him. Certainly, although he was extremely intelligent, Shiro Ishii seems to have lacked empathy towards his fellow human beings. 'As a student, Ishii seemed to have had personality problems: more succinctly, he created problems for others. He was pushy, inconsiderate, and selfish.'[2] He was also callous, and he was driven, which made for an interestingly lethal combination when such a man was placed within the Imperial Japanese Army, one of history's most brutal fighting machines. 'Ishii was a mass of paradoxes; loud and rude, yet also a skilled social and career climber; an ardent nationalist and a devoted scientist, but a wild partygoer too.'[3] It was unusual to find such an overt social climber in Japanese society. 'In a society where Confucian-rooted respect for superiors and a strong consciousness of hierarchy dictates boundaries of behavior, Ishii's forward drive ran roughshod over protocol.'[4] One of his 'debased proclivities' was sleeping with prostitutes who were under sixteen-years-old. Author Daniel Barenblatt has labelled Ishii a 'highly functioning sociopath', and this seems to be a fair assessment of the man in light of his later notorious activities.

One of Ishii's first breakthroughs with the army was his invention of a portable water-filtration device that could be used by troops in the field. It would enable Japanese soldiers to take water from previously dangerous places like rivers, ponds and even puddles. Any war in Asia posed the very serious threat of tropical diseases upon the armies of both sides, and Ishii recognised that it was extremely important to use science to improve the health of Japan's soldiers. So confident was Ishii in his device, that in one notorious incident he urinated into the filter during a demonstration for Emperor Hirohito and then offered the resulting clean water to him to drink. The Emperor understandably declined, but Ishii was noticed in a very positive way. In another stunt later in his career in 1937, Ishii went to the home of Finance Minister Korekiyo Takahashi. On gaining admittance to the house,

Ishii went straight into the kitchen carrying a flask of cultured cholera bacteria. Unless Takahashi immediately granted him a large appropriation to secretly fund BW research, Ishii threatened to pour the contents of the flask all over the kitchen. Takahashi called Ishii's bluff and refused, but swiftly changing tack, the crazed scientist staged a twenty-four hour sit-in, driving the Minister to distraction with his constant badgering until the old man relented and granted Ishii 100 million yen in secret funding. From this grant came the financial support that eventually led to the creation of Unit 731.

Ishii did do some good things before the moral vacuum of Unit 731. Apart from the water-filtration device, in 1924 he was part of a groundbreaking research team who managed to identify a deadly disease subsequently known to science as Japanese B Encephalitis that killed 3,500 people on the island of Shikoku. In a completely different area, Ishii had first demonstrated an interest in using humans as test subjects. As a young army captain in 1927, shortly before his conversion to BW weapons research, Ishii and a colleague had written a very well-received academic article on their research into treating gonorrhea patients. However, the research methodology may have been the catalyst that led Ishii into the field of human experimentation, for the two doctors actually deliberately caused fever in patients through transplanted cells in order to treat the gonorrhea and ultimately to heal the patients. Between 1928 and 1930 Ishii conducted a self-financed world tour, interviewing all of the leading scientists who knew anything about BW research around the globe. His arrival back in Japan was fortuitous, for the political climate had shifted towards the military, and for an ambitious army doctor like Ishii, the rapid advancement of his career became a definite possibility.

In 1928 Japanese agents had attempted to destabilise the northern Chinese province of Manchuria by assassinating the ruling warlord. It was, as with so many 'regime changes' in our own lifetimes, primarily about resources and money. China at this time had no really effective central government. A group of competing warlords, mostly former generals, had controlled the country since the breakdown of the first republic created by Dr. Sun Yat-sen after the last imperial dynasty, the Manchu or Qing, had been overthrown in 1912. A former Imperial general named Yuan Shi-kai had declared himself emperor, but although his reign was measured only in days, the resulting political instability had led to the central government's collapse and the rise of warlordism in the provinces. This meant that China was to all intents and purposes one great big financial opportunity. The British had controlled Hong Kong since the victorious conclusion of the First Opium War in 1842 and they dominated China's most important commercial city, Shanghai, ruling it behind a consortium of business and municipal entities alongside the United States and France. The entire east coast of China was dotted with foreign concessions inside the port cities, meaning that most of the nation's trade was in the hands of foreign business concerns. China was independent in name only. Japan already controlled Manchuria's Liaodong Peninsula (known as the 'Kwantung Leased Territory'), which had been ceded to them by the defeated Russians in 1905 at the conclusion of a short war between the two nations, and Japan also controlled all of the Korean peninsula and the island of Formosa (now Taiwan) off China's coast. Other Japanese territories were the Marshall, Caroline, Marianas and Pescadores Islands in the Pacific, and the port city of Tsingtao (now Qingdao) in China which they had been awarded from a defeated Germany in 1918. It appeared to many of Japan's military leaders that the time had come to take over the rest of Manchuria, a region that is extremely rich in fossil fuels and minerals and packed, then as now, with cheap labour.

The 1928 assassination of the Manchurian warlord brought down the Japanese prime minister's government when it was revealed by the press, and in its place, a more right wing and militarist cabinet met. The Imperial Army saw the Soviet Union as Japan's greatest enemy, and by seizing Manchuria, the Japanese could push their borders north into Mongolia and Siberia, with the eventual aim of conquering the Soviet Far East. They had not reckoned on a determined Red Army and a brilliant Soviet general named Georgy Zhukov who stopped their invasion attempt in its tracks ten years later.

By the mid-1930s, Japan was in the throes of an ultra-nationalist revolution with democracy slowly being pushed out of mainstream politics as reactionary elements in the military and philosophical circles loudly pointed out the inequalities of British and American 'imperialistic' attitudes towards Japan. The Imperial Army followed an ultra-nationalist, quasi-fascist political doctrine known as *Kodaha* (Imperial Way Faction), that had its genesis in the 1920s as a disparate alliance of nationalist groups formed among army officers and had eventually, by the early 1930s, coalesced into one group. Shiro Ishii and his protégés were all adherents, not to mention his many powerful patrons.

Imperial Way was dedicated to establishing the army as the real political power in Japan, either by winning democratic elections, or by more direct methods. Either way, the aim was the establishment of nothing less than a military dictatorship and the expansion of the burgeoning Japanese empire. The Imperial Japanese Navy, though equally nationalistic, followed a different course and made emperor worship its creed. There was considerable tension and distrust between the army and the navy in the follow up to the Second World War and throughout the conflict. The plotters suffered setbacks as well as some stunning victories.

The Great Depression, coupled with early confrontations in China, stirred the ultra-nationalists to take the lead in Japanese foreign policy. Those who stood in the way of the ultra-nationalists' goals often paid a high price. In 1930 Prime Minister Osachi Hamaguchi successfully challenged the military radicals in the army and navy and managed to get the London Naval Conference treaty ratified by the Japanese parliament. The treaty limited the size of Japan's rapidly expanding fleet and maintained the power balance in the Far East with the Royal Navy and United States Navy remaining bigger than the IJN, but in parity with each other.[5] Many ultra-nationalists saw the treaty as an insult to Japan and a reflection of the prevalent racist attitudes of Westerners towards the Japanese people. In November 1930 a would-be assassin wounded Hamaguchi. In 1931 a military coup was planned in Tokyo but it was abandoned at the last minute. The following year naval officers actually assassinated new Prime Minister Tsuyoshi Inukai in the hope of forcing the government to declare martial law, a move that would have placed the military in effective control of the nation. But their plot also failed.

In order for Shiro Ishii's scientific ideas to become reality he needed powerful patrons, and these he began to collect in the new militarist environment in Japan. Ishii first convinced the new Defence Minister, General Sadao Araki, of the necessity of BW research, claiming that his world tour had shown him that many other nations were doing the same thing – and illegally. Major

The Seeds of Death

General Tetsuru Nagata was another early patron. He was an army commander in Manchuria. The Japanese had stationed small numbers of troops in the province for a decade, protecting the main Japanese economic asset in the region – the Russian-built South Manchurian Railway – from bandit attacks in an unstable China. Two of Nagata's subordinates, Colonel Seishiro Itagaki and Lieutenant-Colonel Kenji Ishiwara, hatched a plan to bring about full Japanese control in Manchuria in 1931. They favoured invading and occupying Manchuria and replacing the government with either a Japanese colonial administration or a local puppet regime. They decided to act by sabotaging a section of the South Manchurian Railway near Liutiao Lake and then blaming local Chinese troops. This would give the Japanese Kwantung Army the pretext it needed to occupy the rest of the province, claiming to the rest of the world that they were simply protecting Japanese economic interests in the region. Itagaki, who was Chief of the *Kempeitai* Intelligence Section of the Kwantung Army, led the operation. The *Kempeitai* was Japan's military police, a powerful and feared organisation with some parallels with the German Gestapo and SS Security Police, and the Soviet NKVD – though with a much broader remit.

The Manchurian adventure was a classic 'false flag' intelligence operation of the sort the *Kempeitai* was well-trained to conduct, and it worked perfectly. On 18 September 1931, a small bomb exploded beside the railway track, causing only superficial damage. The next morning Japanese troops attacked the local Chinese garrison which was under strict orders not to resist, and put it to flight. The Chinese did not fight back, believing that this would have led to all-out war and an even bigger disaster for their country. By that evening, Japanese troops had captured the most important city in the region, Mukden (now called Shenyang), for the cost of only two Japanese soldiers killed. Five hundred Chinese troops had been slaughtered during the assault. In spite of the high casualties, Chinese leader Chiang Kai-shek continued to order no resistance to the Japanese, but because of the poor state of communications some Chinese commanders did order their troops into action. Either way, within five months of the so-called 'Mukden Incident' all of Manchuria was under Japanese occupation, and a hesitant Chinese resistance had been swept aside.

Ishii's most helpful mentor was Colonel Chikahiko Koizumi. The much older Koizumi had been involved in chemical warfare research since 1918, and he soon realised that he and Ishii shared the same vision of using chemical and BW weapons to further Japan's nationalistic goals abroad. Koizumi was very well connected with the army's top brass and counted future Japanese Prime Minister and Minister of War Hideki Tojo among his closest friends. In 1930 Koizumi tried to persuade the High Command to reinstitute the army's chemical weapons programme which had been suspended since Japan signed the Geneva Convention in 1925. That same year, he managed to have Ishii promoted to major and made chairman of the department of immunology at Tokyo Army Medical College.

Away from his training and lecturing duties, Ishii and a small team of fellow scientists began to privately culture lethal bacilli in their laboratory, such as bubonic plague, cholera, typhoid and anthrax. In 1931 Koizumi secured funding for Ishii's work, though at this time Ishii was working to create vaccines to protect Japanese troops in the field, rather than to create weapons to deliberately spread deadly pathogens among the enemy. Such was his success, that Ishii's research facility was moved into a two-storey building in 1932 and renamed the 'Epidemic Prevention Laboratory'. At the same time, the army reactivated its dormant chemical warfare unit. By the mid-1930s Japan was manufacturing large numbers of artillery shells containing chlorine, phosgene and mustard gas – clearly with an eye to their deployment in China or the Soviet Union.

The Manchurian situation had become the most important foreign policy problem that the Japanese faced in the 1930s. The Japanese were determined that Manchuria was going to become a state that existed solely to assist the Japanese economy. With its abundant natural resources, the occupied province was soon dubbed 'Japan's lifeline'. As Japan lacked oil and coal deposits in any significant quantities, Manchuria became vital to sustaining not only the Japanese civil economy, but also the rapid expansion of the Imperial Army and Navy. To protect its new territory, the Japanese had in place the 61,000-man Kwantung Army, a force that later grew considerably in size and power. In 1933 – the same year Adolf Hitler became German chancellor – a rather impotent League of Nations condemned Japan's seizure of Manchuria, but the Japanese delegate simply walked out of the meeting after a short speech in which he decried the hypocrisy of the Western Powers who had extensive colonies of their own throughout Asia, and Japan formally withdrew from the League. The last legal constraint placed upon Japan by the international community thus removed, Japan set about re-engineering Manchurian society. Japan had become, to use a modern phrase, a 'rogue state'.

Lieutenant-Colonel Kenji Ishiwara, an Ishii adherent and one of the chief plotters of the 'Mukden Incident', wrote that in his opinion the people of the new Japanese empire in Asia were to be divided thus: 'The four races of Japan, China, Korea and Manchuria will share a common prosperity through a division of responsibilities: Japanese, political leadership and large industry; Chinese, labour and small industry; Koreans, rice; and Manchus, animal husbandry.'[6] Manchuria was the Japanese *lebensraum*, or 'living space', to borrow a term from Nazi empire-building vocabulary. In 1932 the Japanese had legalised their seizure of Manchuria by turning it into a puppet-state they called 'Manchukuo'. Less than two years later, the last Emperor of China, Aisin-Gioro Pu Yi, was installed as Emperor of Manchukuo. Bearing a striking resemblance to Emperor Hirohito, Pu Yi had lost the throne of China in 1912 but he had not been ejected from the Forbidden City in Beijing until 1924. After kicking his heels in Western concessions in China and desperate for a regal role, Pu Yi, a Manchurian of the Qing Dynasty, allowed himself to be installed as leader by the Japanese. This collaboration would make sure that he would face severe punishment after the war from the new communist Chinese government.

In 1936 a group of young Japanese army officers, all adherents of the Imperial Way Faction, launched another coup attempt in Tokyo, killing several prominent politicians in the process. But they also failed to bring the military to full power and they were arrested and later executed. However, the idea still remained of wanting to challenge the Western imperialist nations by forging a large Japanese empire in Asia. The Japanese felt more isolated than ever after withdrawing from the League of Nations after their violent occupation of Manchuria, and their newspapers railed against the 'unfair' treatment the nation was receiving from the Western Powers, who themselves had often resorted to similar displays of military force when carving out their own empires. In this, the Japanese were perfectly correct. The Japanese militarists viewed the international outcry as double standards and racism against a rising Asian power. At home, many ordinary Japanese began to agree with them, and a general feeling that the International Community was unfairly ostracizing Japan soon found widespread support among the masses. This sense of isolationism would find its perfect outlet in the thirst for conquest and dominion beyond the shores of the Sacred Islands. The 'Imperial Way' and its friends had triumphed, but in so doing they would drag their nation to the very point of complete destruction.

With the establishment of firm rule in Manchukuo, Ishii immediately grasped the opportunities to be afforded by establishing a research facility there. Secret human experimentation would be possible for the first time, with the approval of the Imperial Army and the direct assistance of the *Kempeitai* Military Police. 'Members of the *kenpeitai* [sic] were under orders of the army, and were specially selected for their rigid, oppressive, and unyielding personalities. They were given such jobs as catching spies and interrogating suspects, and were authorized to use torture if they were so inclined.'[7] The widespread use of torture by the Japanese military at this time was officially sanctioned. 'The merest fact that someone had been arrested signalled guilt to the Kempeitai, the Japanese legal system of the period placing no stock in the concept 'innocent until proven guilty' or other Western liberal traditions ... Essentially, if you were arrested by the Kempeitai your fate was usually already sealed.'[8] Through such methods would the *Kempeitai* find Ishii's human test subjects.

In Shiro Ishii's mind he was a patriotic servant of the Japanese state. 'He remained a dedicated medical professional who held true to a vision of total military supremacy through the study of and experiments in microbiology,'[9] writes Barenblatt. Ishii's 'vision' was to take the lives of hundreds of thousands of innocent people over the coming decade as science was allowed to run riot without any legal or moral boundaries. The consequences for the peoples of Manchuria and China were catastrophic.

Chapter 2

Paris of the Orient

We heard rumours of people having blood drawn in there, but we never went near the place. We were too afraid.

Chinese witness to the Zhongma Fortress, 1936

Seven men stood in the rain, their bare feet sinking into the mud outside of the poor Manchurian peasant's house. The men, all Chinese or Manchurian, were dressed in rags and their ankles were shackled with old-fashioned leg irons. They were shaking with cold and fright. The family inside the house was terrified by these strange visitors. 'My brother grabbed an axe to defend us,' recalled a witness, 'but when he heard their story he put down the axe. We took the men to a cave on the east side of the house, and started breaking off the shackles.'[1] The secret of Shiro Ishii's human experimentation programme was suddenly, and startlingly, out, but how it managed to leak out to the general population is the story of the genesis of Unit 731 – Japan's murder factory in China.

If the Chinese city of Shanghai was known in the 1930s as the 'Whore of the Orient', then the great northern city of Harbin was the nation's Paris. When the Japanese occupied Manchuria in 1931 they inherited a provincial capital that was more European than Asian in character, architecture and style. When the brutal civil war had drawn to a close in Russia in 1922 after the Bolshevik Revolution, tens of thousands of White Russians, who had been the loyal supporters of Tsar Nicholas II and the Romanov family, fled for their lives to Siberia. From the white hell of Siberia they crossed the border into Manchuria. Many thousands had continued south to wash up in China's most cosmopolitan city, Shanghai, and even today the onion domes of former Russian Orthodox churches stand among the glass skyscrapers downtown. In Harbin, a huge Russian cathedral dominates the cityscape. Many of the streets have the lingering air of St. Petersburg about them, and although the Russian émigrés are long gone, the European flavour of the city still remains in places.

In the early 1930s Harbin was home to over 60,000 Russians. There were universities and a thriving café society similar to pre-war Vienna, and as an exuberant artistic community. As well as the Russians, there were 6,000 Jews in Harbin. Sitting at the confluence of all of the major railway lines in Manchuria, Harbin then, as now, was a polluted and heavily-industrialized city, and at the time was crucial to Japanese economic interests in the region. But once you left the towns and cities, Manchuria was an under-developed, almost feudal, land of rolling grass prairies and high mountains which suffered from an alarmingly bitter Arctic winter and roasting summer. Many writers have drawn the succinct parallel between 1930s Manchuria and the American West in the second half of the nineteenth century. Essentially, Manchuria was the land of opportunity in Asia; a wild and untamed frontier land where fortunes could be made.

Once the Imperial Army had gained full control of the province, millions of Japanese settlers flooded into Manchukuo hoping to export Japanese culture to this most significant new colony. Many came seeking their fortunes. Huge natural resources, an abundant and pliant local labour force, and friendly economic policies made many Japanese businessmen extremely wealthy. It was now the turn of Dr. Shiro Ishii to export something quite different to Manchukuo – BW weapons research. Ishii did not come seeking cheap labour, but free human test subjects drawn from amongst the local populace. Far from the prying eyes of journalists, Ishii and the Imperial Army speedily established the terrible precursor of Unit 731 after an initial false start.

Ishii's first research facility was located in an industrial suburb of Harbin. The Imperial Army gave him a former saké distillery and an adjoining row of shops. These unlikely buildings were speedily transformed into a scientific complex by Ishii's 300-man team. The problems with the location and the site were security and secrecy. The area was densely populated and the main research building was too small. In a sinister move, Ishii demanded that the army provide him with a complex big enough to have its own prison and where he could keep his human guinea pigs under carefully-controlled and monitored scientific standards. The new facility required good communications links with Harbin, but also it had to be far enough away from the main population so as not to arouse suspicion amongst it. The army suggested a small village called Beiyinhe (pronounced 'Bay-yin-her') located around eighty miles southeast of Harbin. A railway line connected it with the city, and army engineers set about building a complex next to a farm close to the village using local labour. Many of the surrounding region's Manchurian inhabitants would find themselves hauled off to Ishii's new laboratories by a *Kempeitai* Military Police detachment based at the site and whose express task was to provide human test subjects for the Japanese scientists.

On 1 August 1936, Ishii, now a lieutenant colonel, was appointed Chief of the Kwantung Army Anti-Epidemic Water Supply and Purification Bureau. This grandiose title was actually a cover for what he and his men were researching, but a clever cover nonetheless. Ishii had been appointed because he 'already was stationed in Manchuria and continued to enjoy excellent connections both with the top echelon within the Kwantung Army and at military headquarters in Tokyo.'[2] Although only a mid-level army officer – the equivalent in rank of a battalion commander in today's British Army – Ishii was more powerful and influential than many generals. 'The Water Purification Bureau was an ideal cover for Ishii. No one could question the value of military units that provided drinkable water to the armed forces,' notes Sheldon H. Harris. 'Ultimately, eighteen or more Water Purification branches proliferated in Manchuria and in China proper. All of the units were under the direct control of Ishii ... And virtually every one of the units at one time engaged in secret BW research using human subjects.'[3]

Ishii's new research facility at Beiyinhe was named the 'Togo Unit' and was placed under the command of Mukden Incident co-conspirator Lieutenant-Colonel Ishiwara. A huge force of labourers, working as mentioned under Japanese Army engineers, set to work building what the local Chinese soon named the Zhong Ma Fortress. An area of 500 square metres was cleared and local inhabitants' houses and shops were ruthlessly demolished. Then a large castle keep-like building rose up in the centre of the site, surrounded by a ten-foot high earthen wall that encompassed approximately one hundred more assorted buildings; the whole complex being surrounded by an electrified fence. Guard towers fitted with machine guns and searchlights were placed around the perimeter. A road running over a drawbridge through some impressive-looking metal gates gave access to the complex. A large *Kempeitai* detachment provided the sentries, as well as mounting roving patrols through the outlying areas around the Fortress. Anyone who was foolish enough to venture too close to the facility without permission was immediately shot. Like the slaves who built the Pharaoh's tombs in Ancient Egypt, large numbers of Chinese labourers who constructed the place were secretly murdered to prevent details of the facility from ever leaking out.

Adjacent to the Fortress, the Japanese built an airstrip where military aircraft both from Japan and all over Manchuria, came to and went from, regularly. Any porters or workmen who entered the Fortress had to wear baskets over their heads to severely limit their vision. The local area was naturally soon alive with gossip about what the Japanese were doing inside the perimeter wall. People disappeared inside the gates and were never seen again. No-one believed the Japanese line that it was a water purification station or a lumber mill; the security arrangements were simply too elaborate.

Ishii's research was, for the first time, designed to produce weaponised pathogens that could be used against Japan's enemies. In the mid-1930s the Japanese Army had identified two specific enemies. Firstly there was the Chinese. Most of the policy makers in Japan's military saw China as the ultimate prize and wanted to invade and occupy its east coast provinces – the richest in the country – and destroy their blood enemies into the bargain. The Chinese Army, though large, was no match for the technologically superior, better-trained and motivated Imperial Japanese Army, and the average Japanese soldier was ideologically stronger and more focused than his Chinese peasant conscript counterpart. The second potential enemy was the Soviet Union, whose armed forces were in an entirely different category from China's. Japan's occupation force in Manchukuo, the Kwantung Army, was forced to cast uneasy glances over its shoulder from time-to-time at the province's northern border. Some Japanese generals clung to an outdated notion of invading the Soviet Far East as Japanese forces had done in 1918 in support of Allied efforts to defeat Bolshevism. At that time, Japanese forces had managed to capture the Soviet city of Vladivostok before finally withdrawing permanently in 1922. But most Japanese generals realised that the Soviet Red Army was now an entirely different proposition. It is an intriguing historical question to think what could have happened if Japan had invaded the Soviet Far East in June 1941 in concert with the German *Blitzkrieg* into European Russia. The entire outcome of the war would probably have been different. However, for the time being, the Japanese and Soviets maintained an uneasy peace. Many officers knew that Ishii's new weapons could have shifted the balance for Japan against either of their proposed foes.

At Beiyinhe, Ishii and the Togo Unit were, for the first time in human history, given the power to perform any kind of experiment that they wished on live human test subjects. These doctors could indulge their curiosity without any fear of censure or punishment. A decade later, when Nazi doctors were given the same powers, they also decided to use humans in the same way that animals had traditionally been used for laboratory experiments. Beiyinhe was the first, long before camps like Auschwitz or Dachau or Mauthausen had even been thought of. Ishii decided to tailor his research to the potential requirements of the Imperial Army. He was particularly interested in diseases such as bubonic plague, which occurred naturally in northern China, posed a danger to Japanese troops, and was a potential weapon against their enemies. Water and food-borne diseases like cholera, typhoid and dysentery were studied aggressively, and dysentery in particular became an important field of research after the Japanese advance into Southeast Asia in 1941–42. It was to figure prominently in later experiments that were conducted on American, British, and Australian prisoners-of-war at Mukden and Tokyo.

Other bacterial diseases studied at Beiyinhe were glanders (a disease found in horses and humans), anthrax and smallpox. An on-site prison at Beiyinhe housed between five hundred and six hundred all-male test subjects, all of whom were aged below forty. The prisoners were kept shackled all the time, but they were well fed, clean and allowed to exercise every day. This was because the Japanese doctors wanted healthy human test subjects to destroy through their experiments. At this stage, all of the prisoners were either Chinese or Manchurians who had been selected by the *Kempeitai*. The criterion for being sent to the Togo Unit was relatively simple: Ishii used political prisoners, bandits and common criminals. *Kempeitai* officers would go through lists of prisoners in their charge, select those who matched the criteria laid down by Ishii, and ship them off. The life expectancy of a prisoner at Beiyinhe was about thirty days, so a large number of prisoners were sent there every month. Major Tomio Karasawa, an army surgeon and mid-level manager who was to later serve with Unit 731 and who provided evidence about the use of Allied prisoners-of-war in human experiments, told his Soviet interrogators in 1945: 'Ishii told me that he had experimented on cholera and plague on the mounted bandits of Manchuria during the winter of 1933–34 and discovered that plague was effective.'[4]

Every two or three days a minimum of 500 cubic centimeters of blood was taken from each patient, rendering many of them extremely weak. Daniel Barenblatt, in *A Plague Upon Humanity*, cites cases where doctors carried out experiments into how much blood could be drained from a human before the patient died. Vivisection experiments were conducted, including the removal of internal organs from live patients; the surgeries being performed without the benefit of anaesthetic because doctors correctly deduced that the drugs would interfere with their research results. Out of curiosity, some of the doctors tried many different forms of lethal experiments, often just testing what the human body could stand. Most of the prisoners at Beiyinhe died from the diseases which were injected into them, or on the operating table as Japanese army surgeons opened them up to study how the diseases affected their internal organs.

Although not much is known about exactly what went on at Beiyinhe (largely because the Japanese destroyed so many of their records in 1945) some eye-witness testimony has survived. Lieutenant General Saburo Endo was one of many high-level army guests who were invited to visit the Togo Unit at Beiyinhe. Endo recorded what he witnessed in his diary on 16 November 1933:

> With Colonel Ando and Lieutenant Tachihara I visited the Transportation Company Experimental Station [the covername of the Togo Unit] and observed experiments ... The Second Squad was responsible for poison gas, liquid poison;

the First Squad electrical experiments. Two bandits were used. 1. Phosgene gas – 5 minute injections of gas into a brick-lined room; the subject was still alive one day after inhalation of gas; critically ill with pneumonia. 2. Potassium Cyanide – the subject injected with 15mg of it; lost consciousness approximately 20 minutes later. 3. 20,000 volts – several jolts of that voltage not enough to kill the subject. 4. 5,000 volts – several jolts not enough; after several minutes of continuous currents, was burned to death.[5]

In August 1934 a prisoner surnamed Li managed to overpower his Japanese guard and grab his keys. Li then freed about forty of his fellow captives, and although their legs remained shackled, with their free hands they started to climb the perimeter wall. A heavy summer downpour had knocked out the facility's electricity, which meant that the perimeter fence was no longer live and the searchlights were out of action. As an alarm klaxon sounded, the Chinese and Manchurian men scrambled up the ten-foot high walls and climbed over the barbed wire at the top. Alerted to the breakout, *Kempeitai* guards managed to shoot down about ten escapees as they climbed the wall or ran off outside, and many more were recaptured in the following hours or succumbed to exposure. Seven men managed to stay free and these men began to tell their horrific stories to local people.

Before very long, the secret of the Togo Unit was well known throughout the region and Ishii was forced to shut the facility and relocate operations to somewhere more secret. He chose a small outlying suburb area of Harbin known as Pingfan, a place that now lives on in infamy as the home of Unit 731. Incredibly, even though seven of the prisoners who escaped from Beiyinhe spoke in detail about what was occurring at the site, the Chinese Nationalist government took no notice. This indifference would prove to have far-reaching consequences once Japan decided to invade the rest of China in 1937.

By mid-1935 the entire test complex at Beiyinhe had been abandoned and razed to the ground. No trace remains today of Unit 731's malignant parent. In 1936 Emperor Hirohito became directly involved in Japan's BW programme. In fact, the Imperial Family was to have frequent and secret dealings with Unit 731 throughout the course of its operation, something that is not widely known. Hirohito personally ordered an expansion of the size of the Togo Unit and its integration into the Kwantung Army proper. The Emperor's command was printed and circulated to army officers in Manchuria so that Japan's BW programme in the region was no longer a closely guarded secret – at least amongst the Japanese military. With the imperial order came an expansion in the personnel size of the Togo Unit; from 300 at Beiyinhe to at least a thousand scientists, researchers and technicians at the unit's new home outside of the village of Pingfan, twenty-six kilometres southwest of Harbin.

Pingfan was quite isolated, but close to the South Manchurian Railway. The Japanese Army cleared an enormous six-square-kilometre area, forcibly relocating local peasants and knocking down their houses. An airstrip was constructed adjacent to the complex and the new test facility was surrounded by a moat, electric fences and guardhouses. The airspace over the complex was restricted and included a standing air patrol over Pingfan with orders to shoot down, without warning, any aircraft that strayed too close.[6] Local people were not allowed, on pain of death, to approach the facility. Ishii's new kingdom would take three years to construct, but medical experiments were begun even before all of the buildings were completed. No expense was spared – with a virtually unlimited budget available from the army, Ishii was able to equip his laboratories with the latest and best facilities that were the envy of similar facilities back in Japan. He would use his budget to attract many of the brightest and best Japanese scientists from universities back home who were thrilled to be able to experiment on humans without any legal restrictions. It is a sad fact that many of Japan's leading post-war scientists had, at one time or another, been involved with Unit 731, though many successfully concealed this fact from the media and historians.

The *Kempeitai* was again placed in charge of finding human test subjects, and they used the well-stocked prisons of Harbin to fill trains with political prisoners and other 'anti-Japanese' suspects, and shipped them off to Pingfan. If they ran short of prisoners they simply rounded up innocent people from the streets. About six hundred men, women and children, including infants, were held inside the prison at Unit 731 at any one time, but because of the high turnover of test subjects, many thousands were required each year to keep the place fully stocked for the scientists. The prison was not some grim mediaeval dungeon, but an up-to-date facility designed to keep the inmates healthy until they were required for experiments. 'Cells were either single- or multiple-occupancy, and were arranged side-by-side, each with its window facing the corridor... Each cell had a flush toilet to maintain cleanliness, a wooden floor, and concrete walls heavier than necessary, probably built with recollections of the escape at Zhongma... Central heating and cooling systems, and a well-planned diet, protected the health of the prisoners to ensure that the data they produced was valid. Poor living conditions or the presence of other disease germs could confuse results.'[7]

Curious locals were fed the story that Pingfan was simply a lumber mill – though only the most gullible believed this lie. Who ever heard of a lumber mill with its own airstrip, a deadly security perimeter and armed guards? The Japanese used the term *'maruta'* – a word that means 'log' in Japanese – when discussing the prisoners. Dr. Ishii's inaugural address to his staff in autumn 1936 revealed clearly the work that the scientists and doctors would be undertaking at Pingfan. His words were unequivocal and are worth reprinting here in full:

> Our God-given mission as doctors is to challenge all varieties of disease-causing micro-organisms; to block all roads of intrusion into the human body; to annihilate all foreign matter resident in our bodies and to devise the most expedient treatment possible. However, the research work upon which we are now to embark is the complete opposite of those principles, and may cause us some anguish as doctors.
>
> Nevertheless I beseech you to pursue this research based on the dual thrill of One: as a scientist to exert efforts to probe for the truth in natural science and research into, and discovery of, the unknown world and Two: as a military person, to successfully build a powerful military weapon against the enemy.[8]

Facilities built included a vast administration building, a guard house, arms magazine, barns for test animals, stables, many laboratory buildings of different sizes and uses, an autopsy/dissecting building, a laboratory for frostbite experiments which was capable of operating year round, and a huge farm producing fresh fruit for the staff, as well as greenhouses that were used in plant BW experiments, a power plant, and a crematorium to dispose of human and animal bodies.[9] In size, it rivalled the vast Auschwitz-Birkenau concentration camp complex built by the Germans in Poland. The Pingfan facility, as well as being a fully equipped human and animal-testing laboratory, was also an extremely well-appointed home for the large community of scientists and their families who lived at the site. The dormitories were comfortable, and the site included restaurants, a bar, and a school for scientists' children, cinema, swimming pool, gardens, library, recreational fields, a Shinto temple and even a Geisha house.[10] 'It was like a resort spa enveloped in a biomedical death camp,' writes Daniel Barenblatt, 'a shocking expression of human inequality.'[11] However, the sole purpose of the facility was to develop lethal BW weapons. That was why the Japanese government funded the facility so lavishly.

Four different types of sentries guarded the Unit 731 facility. The Kwantung Army police, which in turn received support from the Quisling Chinese Gendarmerie, supported the *Kempeitai*, and of course, the ordinary Imperial Army protected the local environs and provided the anti-aircraft batteries and aircraft. A detail of 750 local peasants provided a core force of labourers at the site. They had no human rights and a great many perished.

Before we turn our attention to the POW camp that the Japanese mysteriously established at Mukden, it will help our understanding of what has been alleged to have taken place at Mukden if we first delve a little deeper into the house of horrors at Pingfan to comprehend what the Japanese doctors were interested in. One finds only misery and death at Pingfan, and on a scale that is often difficult to comprehend. Certainly, any examination of Ishii's evil empire is not advised for the weak-stomached or overly imaginative – it is the stuff of nightmares.

Chapter 3

Blood Harvest

No writer of fiction, from the sublime medieval poet Dante Alighieri, to Gothic novelists such as Mary Wollstonecraft Shelley and Robert Louis Stevenson, or modern-day Hollywood-Hong Kong hack science-fiction screenwriters, could possibly rival the real-life misdeeds of Ishii and his fellow researchers. The charnel house that Ishii created at Ping Fan and its satellite facilities throughout Manchuria and China proper is, arguably, inconceivable by the most fertile fictive imagination.

Sheldon H. Harris, Author of *Factories of Death*[1]

Pingfan was an impressive piece of engineering, and it demonstrated absolutely the Japanese will to make BW weapons development a top priority. In order to build it, Shiro Ishii had ordered the razing of eight Manchurian villages in total. With a perimeter fence encompassing a camp of several square miles, the Pingfan facility contained not only well-appointed living quarters and staff facilities for the thousands of Japanese researchers and medics who would work there, but also a *Kempeitai* barracks, a prison camp to house test subjects, underground bunkers, dungeons and gas chambers, scientific laboratories and operating theatres. The list is virtually endless. In an eerie precursor to Auschwitz and Belsen, there was, as mentioned, a crematorium used to dispose of prisoners' bodies once medical experiments had been completed. In total, there were about one-hundred-and-fifty structures on the site, many of which have survived to this day due to their solid and expensive construction. In fact, it was this very solidity that prevented the Japanese from erasing all traces of their terrible crimes at Pingfan at the conclusion of the war.

As we have also seen, Unit 731 was an integral part of the Kwantung Army, though the Japanese high command tried to downplay this relationship after the war, and used the disingenuous cover name 'Epidemic Prevention Department' in a vain attempt to explain away its existence, and that of seventeen other similar centres across Asia that are known about. Amazingly, we still do not know the full extent of Unit 731's empire.

Dr. Ishii and his peers were busy developing lethal weapons and conducting inhumane experiments on people; experiments that plumbed the very depths of depravity and sadism, and all in the cause of 'science'. The people who were gathered at Pingfan were men, women, children and infants. They were mostly Chinese, but they also included some Koreans, White Russians and, as we shall see, Allied prisoners-of-war from the United States, Britain and Australia. The Japanese calling the prisoners *maruta*, meaning 'logs', was an in-joke among the staff after the Japanese told the local population that the facility was a lumber mill. It was also an indication of how these men viewed the humans that they experimented upon.

Recent research by Chinese academics at the Harbin Academy of Social Sciences has identified the names of 1,463 people who were secretly sent to Pingfan by the *Kempeitai* for use as human guinea pigs, and a conservative figure of between five thousand and twelve thousand people is the number the Japanese most likely murdered at Unit 731. Ishii believed that the results of the research undertaken at Pingfan would far outweigh the cost in human lives, and the doctors' disregard for their Hippocratic Oath. 'A doctor's God-given mission is to block and treat disease,' Ishii said to his staff of scientists shortly after their arrival, 'but the work on which we are now to embark is the complete opposite of those principles.'[2]

The civilian prisoners who were sent to Pingfan had their files marked 'Special Deportation' by the *Kempeitai* who often added other comments like 'incorrigible', 'die-hard anti-Japanese' and 'of no value or use' when describing the prisoners.[3] The Military Police dehumanised its captives and feeding the laboratories at Pingfan was a useful exercise in ridding Manchukuo (as the

Japanese now called Manchuria) of people it did not like, regardless of whether they had broken the law or not. The 'special deportations' begun on the orders of Ishii on 26 January 1936, as the scientists demanded increasing numbers of human test subjects. In 1941 the facility was officially renamed the 'Epidemic Prevention and Water Purification Department of the Kwantung Army', using the military designation 'Unit 731' for short. It is from this date that the term 'Unit 731' was in common Japanese circulation, though its activities at Pingfan and elsewhere remained above top secret. Support for the experiments being conducted at Pingfan came directly from Japanese universities and pharmaceutical companies in the Home Islands, as well as from the *Kempeitai* and the Japanese government. The work undertaken by Unit 731 was seen as vital to the Japanese war effort, and no expense was spared in making the facilities as up-to-date as possible.

Unit 731 was divided into eight divisions, all under Ishii's overall command. Ishii himself was quickly promoted to the rank of major general, and later to lieutenant general, as his fiefdom increased in size and influence. Division 1 conducted research into bubonic plague, cholera, anthrax, typhoid, and tuberculosis using live human subjects. These were drawn like guinea pigs from a special camp that held around three hundred to four hundred prisoners on site, and was always kept fully stocked by the *Kempeitai*. The life expectancy of prisoners held in this medical prison was measured in just a few weeks at most. Division 2 conducted research into biological weapons that could be used by troops in the field, and concentrated particularly on inventing new devices to release germs and infected parasites – in effect, designing and building biological warfare bombs. Division 3 ran a factory which actually produced artillery shells containing biological agents and was based off-site in the city of Harbin. Division 4 produced other lethal agents, while Division 5 was responsible for training Unit 731 personnel. Divisions 6–8 looked after equipment, medical supplies and camp administration respectively, and these sections did not play a role in murdering people directly.[4]

The kinds of experiments conducted on live human subjects were numerous and terrible. Vivisection was practiced with alacrity by Unit 731 medical staff. No anaesthetics were administered to victims before they were sliced up and dismembered because doctors believed that the drugs would interfere with their research results. Prisoners were infected with various bacteria that the scientists wished to study, and after the resulting disease or infection had progressed, they were vivisected as part of an internal examination. 'The fellow knew that it was over for him, and so he didn't struggle when they led him into the room and tied him down,' recalled a seventy-two-year-old former medical assistant at Unit 731 when interviewed in the 1990s and describing a thirty-year-old Chinese male victim. 'But when I picked up the scalpel, that's when he began screaming.' The horror of the event was simply a routine procedure at Pingfan. 'I cut him open from the chest to the stomach, and he screamed terribly, and his face was all twisted in agony. He made this unimaginable sound, he was screaming so horribly. But then he finally stopped. This was all in a day's work for the surgeons, but it really left an impression on me because it was my first time.'[5]

Allied to Unit 731 were a number of test sites or sub-units located throughout Asia. About eighty miles from Pingfan there was an open-air testing site at Anta. Unit 100 was located at Changchun and was codenamed the 'Wakamatsu Unit'. It was under the command of veterinarian Yujiro Wakamatsu. This unit was dedicated to developing vaccines to protect Japanese livestock and developing lethal animal diseases that could be deployed against Chinese and Soviet livestock. Biological sabotage was an important duty of Unit 100.

In Beijing, the Japanese had established Unit 1855, an experimental branch of Unit 731 with a research facility at Chinan in Hopei Province. Unit 1855 scientists conducted research mainly into bubonic plague and other diseases. In the Chinese capital Nanjing – earlier devastated by Japanese atrocities, looting and vandalism in 1937–38 – Unit 731 maintained another satellite station, Unit Ei-1644, codenamed the 'Tama Unit' after the surname of its commander, which collaborated with Pingfan on many joint projects and experiments. In southern China, at Canton (now Guangzhou) near Hong Kong, the Japanese established Unit 8604 which they codenamed the 'Nami Unit'. This unit was the main rat farm for the Kwantung Army, breeding millions of the rodents for use in biological warfare applications. Also at Unit 8604, the Japanese conducted human deprivation experiments as well as research into water-borne viruses such as typhus and cholera.

And so the list goes on, indicating that Shiro Ishii really had managed to create a biological warfare empire across occupied Asia. Unit 200 was based in Manchuria, and again worked closely with Pingfan on plague research. The Japanese were not seeking a cure for the plague, but rather, were interested in developing new, and considerably more lethal, strains that could be unleashed on the Chinese population. There was also another facility in Manchuria, Unit 571, closely associated with Pingfan, but the site of its headquarters is currently unknown to historians and the nature of the research conducted there remains a mystery to this day. The Mukden Military Hospital, only a few miles from the Mukden POW Camp, was another Unit 731 research centre, and several of the sickest Allied prisoners from the camp were sent there for treatment. Outside of China, Unit 731's tentacles stretched deep into the rest of Asia. The biggest unit was based at the prestigious Raffles Medical University in Singapore. Established in February 1942 shortly after the ignominious British surrender of the colony, Unit 9420 consisted of about a thousand personnel under the command of Major General Masataka Kitagawa and was under the operational day-to-day control of Lieutenant-Colonel Ryoichi Naito. It was divided into two parts: 'Kono Unit' which specialised in research into malaria, and the 'Umeoka Unit' which was interested once again in plagues. Evidence has come to light that Unit 9420 operated another sub-unit in Thailand during the war, but for what purpose it is unfortunately not known, the Japanese having partially destroyed records of their medical research before Allied war crimes investigation teams arrived in September 1945.

General Ishii's empire of death also extended into Japan itself, to the oldest facility located in the southern city of Hiroshima. Here, the Japanese had established their first chemical weapons factory in 1928, manufacturing mustard gas, but it later moved on to producing much more lethal poisons for military usage. During the 1930s the Japanese government ordered the removal of the factory and research facility from all maps of the area to preserve its secrecy and security.

The prisoners at Unit 731 were kept shackled hand and foot at all times to prevent their escape, but they were well fed and exercised regularly, for obvious reasons that also bear some relation to the treatment of American, British and Australian POWs at

Mukden Camp where they were kept much healthier than comparable prisoners in other Japanese prison camps. 'Unless you work with a healthy body you can't get results,'[6] explained one former Japanese member of staff. Prisoners at Pingfan and elsewhere were deliberately infected with various diseases and then dissected while alive so that doctors could observe the results of the diseases on the human body. Men, women and children were used. Other examples included doctors raping female prisoners to make them pregnant, and several months later these same women were dissected and the fetuses removed while they were alive.

Limbs were often amputated to study the effects of bloodloss. Sometimes, Japanese surgeons would reattach the severed limbs to different parts of the body; for example, sewing legs into arm sockets and so on, in horrific Frankenstein experiments. Freezing tests were conducted where limbs were frozen and then amputated, while others were defrosted intact to study the effects of gangrene on live tissue. In fact, this research turned out to be some of the most useful made by Unit 731 and is still informing medical opinion regarding frostbite injuries today. The methods used in the research were, however, extremely cruel and painful. During the winter prisoners were staked out in fields and their bare arms drenched in cold water to accelerate the freezing process. Scientists would strike the arms with a stick to test whether they were frozen – if they heard a hard, hollow sound the freezing was judged to be complete. Defrosting caused the onset of gangrene, as well as intense pain, which was then studied carefully. Once the prisoners had outlived their usefulness they were killed and their bodies disposed of in the camp crematorium.

Some prisoners had their stomachs removed and the oesophagus reattached to the intestines. Others were tied down, and parts of their various organs, such as the brain, liver, kidneys, lungs and so on, were removed. Many of these experiments were conducted on infants who lay screaming for their mothers, their short lives abruptly terminated by doctors who viewed these little children as nothing more than live flesh to play with. The cruelties of the doctors were almost beyond explanation, and suffice to say, to recount them here would not be appropriate. Another story that highlights how cheap a human life was at Unit 731 was when General Ishii one day demanded a human brain to experiment on. A group of *Kempeitai* guards 'grabbed a prisoner and held him down while one of them cleaved open his skull with an axe. The brain was removed and rushed to Ishii's laboratory.'[7]

Dozens of former medical staff employed at Unit 731 remain alive in Japan today, and several have come forward to talk about what they did to prisoners in the name of science. One man, surnamed Kamada, recalled his dissection of a live *maruta* who had been deliberately infected with plague bacteria. 'I inserted the scalpel directly into the log's neck and opened the chest,' stated Kamada. 'At first there was a terrible scream, but the voice soon fell silent.'[8]

Testing the effects of battlefield weapons on live human targets was considered by the Japanese to be very important research, not the least in the area of battlefield medicine. Prisoners were tied to wooden stakes on special ranges and grenades exploded at different distances from them to study the effects. Some prisoners were shot and the resultant wounds examined before the prisoners were killed. Flamethrowers were used on human subjects to test the most effective range for use of the weapon on the battlefield, and other poor souls were taken to the open-air testing facility at Anta and exposed to biological and chemical weapons to test their effects, many of which were dropped from aircraft as the Japanese strove to perfect useable biological warfare bombs.

Disease research was at the centre of Unit 731's operations. Prisoners were told they were receiving vaccinations, when in reality the Japanese deliberately infected them with all sorts of terminal diseases to study their effects on human subjects. Sexual diseases such as syphilis and gonorrhea were passed to males and females via rape and left to fester so that the results could be studied before the patients were executed. Huge numbers of fleas were introduced to infected patients so that the Japanese could breed billions of the infected insects for use in biological warfare bombs. These weapons were later used on the Chinese population. Low-flying Japanese aircraft released special canisters containing plague-infected fleas over Chinese cities including Ningbo in 1940 and Changde in 1941. The resulting disease epidemics killed upwards of four-hundred-thousand Chinese civilians, and were one of the least-known war crimes of the Second World War. In fact, more Chinese died as a result of Unit 731's germ bombs than all of the Japanese killed at Hiroshima and Nagasaki by the atomic bombs combined together. Yet we hear or read remarkably little about these horrendous crimes against humanity, while the world is expected to show a unified respect and sorrow for the sufferings of the Japanese annually. Infections caused by these aerial bombing experiments in China, and others like them, were still killing people in the north of the country in 1948, three years after the war had ended.

Some of the human experiments were bizarre, and initially appeared devoid of medical reason. Prisoners were hung upside down to see how long it would take for them to die. Air was injected into prisoners' arteries to induce fatal blood clots. Horse urine was injected into human kidneys. Of more medical use were the special high-pressure chamber experiments that were conducted as Japan developed jet aircraft in close cooperation with the Germans, whose doctors were also conducting high altitude tests on Jewish prisoners in the concentration camps. Extremes of temperature and their effects on the human body were studied intensively, alongside water and food deprivation experiments, including some that have been well-documented using Allied prisoners-of-war.

The list of ways in which Unit 731 doctors killed their test subjects was long. For example, giant centrifuges were built to test how much G-force the human body could withstand, and these experiments were naturally fatal to the test subjects as the speed was increased and increased. X-ray radiation was administered to prisoners, including lethal doses. The Japanese constructed gas chambers where chemical weapons were tested on live prisoners.[9] The list of atrocities and crimes is nearly endless, and each experiment broke just about every ethic known to medical science as well as to International Law.

Some of the experiments produced no useful scientific data, but many did advance human knowledge. It is a sad fact that when Japanese and German doctors were permitted to do as they pleased with prisoners – in effect to play God – the terrible suffering produced data that was invaluable after the war in developing the weapons of the Cold War and for sending Man into space. Without German and Japanese research into rocketry and the human body's endurance, the United States would never have reached the Moon in 1969. As will be examined later, it was the United States that cynically protected German and Japanese scientists and doctors who had been involved in these crimes against humanity in order to give America the technological edge over the Soviet Union during the Cold War. This is not in dispute. What is in dispute is whether the Japanese in the course of these experiments killed American, British and Australian POWs, and whether the Allied Powers later cynically used the data thus collected and collated for their own ends.

Knowledge of what was happening at Pingfan was widely known throughout the highest echelons of the Japanese government and was officially sanctioned. Even the Imperial Family was familiar with Unit 731's activities. Prince Mikasa, Emperor Hirohito's younger brother, actually toured the Unit 731 facility where he was shown films of Chinese prisoners 'made to march on the plains of Manchuria for poison gas experiments on humans'[10], as he noted in his published memoirs. General Hideki Tojo, who was Prime Minister of Japan and Minister of War for most of the conflict, was so pleased by General Ishii's test results that he saw to it that the Emperor awarded Ishii a high decoration. After the Japanese surrender in August 1945, the Imperial Household Agency, the Japanese government and the military high command all engaged in a furious back-pedaling exercise in an attempt to prevent the Emperor and members of his family from having to personally answer for the war crimes that had been committed by subordinates that had acted on their orders. It was a cover-up that has remained in place to this day, a cover-up that was encouraged and aided by American complicity as agents of the United States intelligence community raced to secure the secrets of Unit 731 for the nation. And in amongst this complicated story there lies the equally disturbing account of the Allied POWs at the Mukden Camp, and their unwitting roles in furthering the insane research of Unit 731.

Chapter 4

The Camp

I was reminded of Dante's Inferno *– abandon hope all ye who enter here ...*

Major Robert Peaty, Mukden Camp, 1942

In the dead of night an American prisoner-of-war suddenly awoke from a fitful sleep. The face peering down at him was Japanese. The hard, almond-shaped eyes looked surprised beneath the field service cap adorned with a yellow star that the young soldier wore. The American felt something tickling him underneath his nose, and he was astonished when the Japanese soldier withdrew a hand that was holding a coloured feather. This surreal scene ended with the Japanese apologising, itself an almost unheard-of event, before he disappeared into the gloom of the unlit wooden barracks. The next day, many of the other POWs in the hut reported similar nocturnal visits by mysterious Japanese soldiers armed with feathers. It was just one night of many when the Japanese would pay surreptitious visits to the hundreds of prisoners living in the Mukden Camp.

There are aspects of the story of the Mukden prisoner-of-war camp that are so different in comparison to what historians know of so many other Japanese prison camps that Mukden can be seen as a special case. A detailed examination of the camp reveals many anomalies that fit in with the hypothesis that the camp had been created by the Japanese and stocked with Allied POWs for some nefarious purpose other than simply to imprison them, or to use them as hard labour. The evidence points to a direct link between

The Camp

what occurred inside the Mukden Camp and the activities of Unit 731 at Pingfan.

Before we begin to examine the evidence of secret medical experiments being carried out at Mukden Camp, we should examine the aspects of the Mukden Camp that are problematic and arouse suspicion as to its purpose. They are as follows: (i) its location in Manchuria; (ii) the number of prisoners it held; (iii) the camp administration; (iv) the behaviour of the Japanese guards towards the prisoners; (v) conditions inside the camp for the prisoners; (vi) the food rations, and; (vii) the large medical facilities that were present. We need to address the startling anomalies that are already clearly shown in the surviving documents and witness statements. Later in this book we will examine actual witness statements and documents from American, British, Russian and Japanese sources that address the question of medical experimentation on Allied POWs at Mukden, but for the time being it is important to clearly identify Mukden's dissimilarity from a standard Japanese POW camp in order to show that the opportunity existed for the Japanese to conduct a secret experimentation programme at the site.

* * *

The Allied POWs who ended up at Mukden came from two completely different locations and from several different armies. The possible reasons for the national composition of the prisoners in the camp will be examined later, for it has some significance if we accept any interference in the camp by Unit 731 doctors. The Americans were shipped in from the Philippines where they had been extremely harshly treated in the prison camps established there for the survivors of the Bataan Death March and Corregidor Island. Their shipment to Mukden was well documented in the secret diary of Private Sigmund Schreiner, a twenty-three-year-old Army Air Corps technician from Connecticut, who had managed to survive the Bataan Death March. On 6 October 1942 several thousand American POWs were assembled at the docks in Manila and herded aboard the Japanese 'hellship' *Totori Maru*, beginning what turned out to be a forty day journey to Mukden in Manchuria. Acting as guards for the journey were about a thousand regular Japanese troops who were being reassigned to a different command in China. The conditions the American prisoners endured, crammed into the hold of the ship bereft of adequate light, food, water and lavatory facilities, were appalling. They were barely able to lie down, such was the overcrowding, and the Japanese also starved them, often handing out only half a loaf of bread each day. Sometimes this was supplemented with Japanese military biscuits or a meal of boiled rice. Schreiner described how bad the accommodations on the ship were: 'The air was foul and the lice situation in a terrific state.'[1]

The Americans were already malnourished from their experiences in prisoner-of-war camps in the Philippines, and many were sick with tropical diseases. The prisoners were assigned only one latrine with space for five men, and dysentery started up among them soon after the voyage began. 'Most of us had diarrhoea and other intestinal diseases,' recalled Private Schreiner. 'The number of cases suddenly started to increase rapidly. The reason for this was finally discovered when someone happened to glance into the water tank and see a pair of dirty shorts floating around.'[2] The tank was cleaned and the eight US Army doctors accompanying the men had a busy time trying to treat the worst affected without any medicine. They were lucky to survive after an American submarine fired two torpedoes at their ship on the first day out – fortunately for everyone concerned the torpedoes missed. The Japanese routinely refused to clearly mark POW transport ships and thousands of Allied prisoners drowned at sea after their ships were sunk by British, American and Dutch submarines that were heavily interdicting Japan's merchant fleet.

The *Totori Maru* made a stop at the Japanese island of Formosa where it was coaled, resupplied and took fresh water on board. Following a short stop in Japan, the ship docked in Pusan, at the tip of the Korean peninsula, on 8 October 1942, and two-thirds of the men remaining aboard were offloaded, de-loused, issued with Japanese clothing and then marched through the city so that the local residents could admire the martial qualities of Japan as the bedraggled and ill Caucasian POWs were ritually humiliated before them.

They were in the main malnourished and diseased upon their arrival at Mukden Camp three days later, after pausing to collect a party of British, Australian and New Zealand prisoners. In contrast, the British and Commonwealth prisoners had been sent

The Camp

direct from the giant Changi Cantonment which was run by the British and Australians themselves with the minimum of interference from the Japanese since the surrender of Singapore in February 1942. This meant that the British and Australian soldiers were in better physical and mental condition than their American comrades on arrival in northern Asia.

The British also benefitted from the strong regimental system that still exists in the British Army; where one's unit becomes one's family and support network, and where one's cap badge is inextricably linked to often hundreds of years of regimental history and tradition that has been instilled into every new recruit. This was something that the Americans lacked to a very large degree, and many senior British officers who were captured at the fall of Singapore and subsequently imprisoned alongside US Army troops in Manchuria, pointedly commented upon this.

The small party of British and Australian POWs who ended up at Mukden were one tenth of the total number who had been shipped out of Singapore on 19 August 1942. Three days earlier 1,000 British and Australian troops had been driven in a huge fleet of requisitioned British trucks from Changi to the Singapore docks. There, they had been loaded aboard a rusting steamer, the 3,821-ton *Fukai Maru*. 'We were allowed one kit bag, one haversack and a pack but no jewellery or indecent photographs,'[3] recalled Corporal Eric Wallwork about the move. The majority of the British prisoners were from 2nd Battalion, The Loyal Regiment (North Lancashire) or the Royal Artillery. The trucks were 'very crowded, each truck carrying 29 men and 1 officer.'[4] The British and Australians soon discovered that their accommodation aboard the *Fukai Maru* was equally overcrowded. After dumping all of their baggage on the quayside so that the Japanese could fumigate it, the men on the ship were forced to 'undress and get into a large and evil-smelling disinfectant bath.' A Senior Officer's Party, made up of the generals, brigadiers and staff colonels captured in Singapore, was given the same treatment. The officers were destined for a new camp in Formosa. The Japanese intended to make examples of them. Lieutenant-General Arthur Percival, British commander-in-chief in Malaya, recalled that after their bath and before embarking on another hellship called the *Tanjong Maru* that was moored beside the *Fukai Maru*, 'we were tested for dysentery and disinfected. The Japanese are great people for tests and inoculations.'[5]

The *Fukai Maru* was fully loaded with 1,000 British and Australian POWs on 16 August 1942. The men were divided between two filthy and vermin-infested holds in the ship. On 19 August the vessel weighed anchor and headed out to sea. On 22 August it anchored again, this time off Cholon Sumyak on the Sumyak River in Malaya, where five other ships including the *Tanjong Maru* joined it. Sailing again the following day, the little convoy arrived at Takao in Formosa on 29 August. The Senior Officer's Party went ashore, as did all of the POWs from the *Fukai Maru* who were put to work for two back-breaking weeks loading the rusting steamer with sacks of bauxite. This meant that their already cramped quarters were made even more unbearable by this additional cargo. Setting sail on the 15 September, at the beginning of the typhoon season, the ship joined another convoy off the Pescadores and headed north into the South China Sea and rough weather.

Conditions for the POWs aboard the ship were less than desirable. The Japanese served only two lean meals per day, at 10am and 4pm, which consisted of boiled rice, thin soup, a few onions and fourteen tins of Irish stew to be shared between the 1,100 POWs aboard. The rough seas only compounded the men's misery, with seasickness added to the rampant dysentery and diarrhoea already doing the rounds. Outrigger latrines were erected along the ship's sides but after these were washed away by heavy waves the sanitary conditions down below were distressing. The men also suffered when the temperature dropped as the ship steamed north. On arrival at Pusan in Korea on 22 September, the holds were fumigated and the prisoners offloaded and inspected by Japanese doctors. Nearly everyone was ill with either beriberi or acute diarrhoea, while the twenty men who were sick with dysentery were removed to a local hospital. On the quayside the *Kempeitai* relieved the POWs of watches, wedding rings and personal photographs, and then forced the men to march all day through the town, where the locals, including school children, were encouraged to jeer and spit at the Allied soldiers. After this final humiliation the POWs were dispatched to various POW camps.

The death rate of Allied POWs in Korea during 1942–43 was 2.7%, a very low figure when compared with other parts of the

The Camp

Japanese Empire. The reason for this was probably because the Japanese wanted the British and Australians in Korea for their propaganda value. Certainly, the prisoners themselves noted the number of visits that they received from Japanese reporters and camera crews. The Red Cross was also allowed easier access to the camps than in other locations. A hundred British and Australian POWs were selected from one camp in Korea and sent into Manchuria, where they joined the American prisoners from the Philippines. For the rest who were left behind, the attitude of the Japanese changed in late 1943. They were sent to a series of increasingly harsh new camps where they were forced to toil in local factories. The death rate rose alarmingly.

We should note at this point the exact number of Allied prisoners who were involved in the relocation to Mukden in Manchuria. Thirty-one officers and 1,962 American enlisted personnel had left Manila aboard the *Totori Maru* on 8 October 1942. During the journey north eleven of these men died onboard the ship, evidence of their poor condition when the journey began and of their general ill treatment and neglect during the course of the journey by their Japanese guards. The Japanese dumped their bodies over the side. On arrival at Takao in Formosa fourteen of the prisoners were off-loaded and taken to a local hospital. The rest continued with the voyage, arriving at the port city of Kobe in Japan where a further sixteen officers and 569 enlisted personnel were transferred to a nearby camp to be used as labour. The remainder of the POWs, under the command of the senior American officer, Major Stanley Hankins of the US Coast Artillery, steamed on to the Korean port of Pusan (now Busan) where one officer and 180 enlisted men were transferred to a local hospital. At this point, the 'British' party (more accurately the 'Commonwealth party'), which consisted of eighty-four British and sixteen Australian and New Zealand soldiers under the command of Major Robert Peaty, Officer Commanding No. 4 Ordnance Store Company, Royal Army Ordnance Corps, joined the American party and entrained for Mukden together before arriving at their final destination on 11 November 1942. Peaty had been captured at the fall of Singapore on 15 February 1942 after his company of 400 men had only recently arrived from Durban in South Africa. He endured the voyage north with a handful of his original unit aboard the *Fukai Maru*.

The choice of Mukden as the site of a POW camp is interesting. It was 350 miles south of Unit 731's main facility near Harbin and many hundreds of miles from the nearest comparable POW camp in China. The American historian Linda Goetz Holmes who wrote an extremely detailed book about the camp, suggested that the main reason why a large group of Allied POWs was brought to the Mukden area was to labour for the Mitsubishi Corporation which owned and operated several businesses nearby. This would make sense, for Mitsubishi, like many other Japanese companies, and similar to famous German enterprises like Siemens, lobbied their respective governments to give them Allied POWs for use as virtual slave labourers. Mitsubishi owned and operated the hell ship that brought the prisoners to Manchuria from Manila, and a mine in Japan where some of them were later dispatched for punishment. The company was basically a war profiteer that was in cahoots with the Japanese government through complex historical relationships, and it was extremely ruthless in its illegal exploitation of Allied POWs as nearly free labour. The camp was also far enough away from Pingfan so as not to arouse any suspicions of an association with Unit 731, but sufficiently close to the Mukden Military Hospital, an out-station that did conduct research for Unit 731. The camp was also nicely isolated from other similar POW centres, but still well connected to the all-important regional transport grid.

The Allied prisoners-of-war arrived at the Mukden Camp together on 11 November 1942. There were, in total, 1,202 Americans, eighty-four Britons and sixteen Australians and New Zealanders. The first camp that they were imprisoned at was a temporary affair created by the Japanese out of a former Chinese barracks complex and located about one mile north of the Mukden city limits. It had originally been constructed just after the turn of the century and was in a poor state of repair. 'I would not keep my garden tools in such a shed,'[6] commented Major Peaty of the accommodation. As with Pingfan, the facility was located next to an airstrip disguised as a dairy farm to protect it from aerial observation or attack, and close to the main railway line to the city of Changchun, where Unit 731 was also operational.

The senior American officer in the camp, Major Hankins, had thirteen other Americans officers assisting him. His British counterpart, Major Robert Peaty, and a handful of Commonwealth

The Camp

junior officers, were responsible for the welfare of the British, Australian and New Zealand parties, but cooperated closely with the Americans. Peaty was a kind of de facto deputy to Major Hankins, who, as the senior officer of the largest national contingent, was also the senior *Allied* officer in the camp. There were also several military doctors among the officer prisoners including Captain Mark G. Herbst of the US Army and Captain Desmond Brennan, 2/3rd Mobile Ambulance Corps, Australian Army Medical Corps. Brennan was one of six Australian officers sent with a large party of other ranks from Changi to Korea onboard the *Fukai Maru* alongside the British. Both Peaty and Brennan kept secret diaries during their time at Mukden detailing how the men were treated, as well as making careful note of the high death rate that took so many American lives during the first few months of imprisonment in Manchuria. Both Major Hankins and Captain Herbst gave detailed reports on their experiences after their liberation in 1945 to the US Department of Defense.

Arriving at such northern latitudes in the depths of the harsh Manchurian winter meant that the prisoners suffered greatly from the elements. They had been shipped from the tropical Philippines and Singapore respectively, straight into the maw of the Chinese winter, when sub-zero winds and snowstorms blow down unchecked from Siberia and Mongolia. The Americans suffered more than the British and Australian prisoners, owing to their poorer physical condition after a hard imprisonment in the Philippines. The British and Australians had been much better off running their own show inside the vast Changi Cantonment. They managed to avoid most of the malnutrition that was endemic inside Japanese-run camps and the casual brutality of their guards who, for the most, were kept well away from the British Commonwealth prisoners. The Japanese took the unusual step of arming local Sikhs – many of them Indian nationalists – and employing them as guards at Changi. It would be an important factor in the survival of the Commonwealth prisoners at Mukden, but it does not entirely explain the huge disparity in the death rates of the different nationalities imprisoned together at the camp.

As the long line of frozen prisoners trudged dejectedly through the gates of the Mukden Camp on 11 November 1942, each man wore Japanese issued winter clothing along with an assortment of uniform odds and ends from their original tropical kit. Japanese guards, their rifles with fixed bayonets held at the port, guarded the flanks and rear of the column as a *tenko* roll-call parade was ordered on the central parade square. Emerging from the warmth of his office the camp commandant, Colonel Matsuyama, strode across the front of the halted ranks of grumbling, shivering, sneezing and coughing POWs. He was followed attentively by his executive officer, Lieutenant Terao, and the chief medical officer, Captain Kawajima. Beneath their soft field service caps the Japanese officers eyed their new charges with suspicion, Matsuyama impatiently tapping one of his high brown jackboots with his sheathed *samurai* sword. After a curt speech of welcome translated from Japanese into English by the army interpreter and peppered with the usual warnings and admonitions for good behaviour, the prisoners fell out and were assigned to their barracks.

At this point in the story we have intimation that Mukden was something quite different from an ordinary run-of-the-mill Japanese prison camp. One of the first clues is the commandant himself, Colonel Matsuyama. Why was such a senior ranking officer put in charge of such a tiny camp? Based on what we know about other Japanese prison camps and civilian internment centres, the Japanese military, owing to their view that POWs and internees were considered to barely exist on the same level as native coolies, normally assigned very junior officers to command large numbers of prisoners. The commandant's rank would reveal much about how a face- and hierarchy-obsessed Asian enemy viewed its charges. For example, the giant Tjideng Ghetto, a vast holding camp for Dutch and British women and children located in a poor area of Batavia (now Jakarta) in the Netherlands East Indies, at its peak occupancy held over ten thousand people. The commandant was a lowly subaltern, Lieutenant Kenichi Sonei, (although he was later promoted to captain). At Batu Lintang Camp in Borneo, a mixed prisoner-of-war and civilian internment camp holding several thousand men, women and children, the commandant held the rank of lieutenant colonel. But Lieutenant-Colonel Tatsuji Suga was also responsible for *all* other prison camps on the whole of Borneo Island and merely had his headquarters at Batu Lintang. When he was frequently away at other camps his second-in-command, a captain, exercised full command duties. Under this system we find another junior officer, Captain Susumi Hoshijima,

The Camp

responsible for three prison camps at Sandakan in northeast Borneo that contained several thousand Australian and British soldiers (who were later murdered on the infamous Sandakan Death March in 1945). The military rank of the Mukden commandant is extremely important because it indicates that the Japanese considered the camp to be special for some unspecified reason. This is confirmed by the fact that when Colonel Matsuyama left his post on 2 December 1942, another full colonel by the name of Genji Matsuda, who held the post until the Japanese surrender, immediately replaced him.

* * *

As mentioned above, a suggested purpose of the Mukden Camp was to house POW workers who would provide labour for a series of Mitsubishi-owned factories that were deliberately located close by. The Allied POWs who ended up at Mukden may have been deliberately requested by the Mitsubishi Corporation so that their labour could assist the company to grow richer, and also to greatly assist the Japanese war effort in the process. It may be that the labour the POWs were forced to undertake was merely coincidental to their real purpose at Mukden – that of guinea pigs for the study of infectious diseases. It was never the intention of the Japanese that the prisoners should sit around idle and making use of them as labourers made perfect sense. They remained in situ for use as test subjects as and when required, but in the meantime also performed important functions for the Japanese war economy. As they were not shipped directly to Unit 731 at Pingfan we can surmise that the Japanese wanted any medical experimentation performed on Caucasian prisoners to be kept low-key. It was an extremely sensitive area after all, and one that required careful handling. Allied POWs were not Chinese peasants and they could not be made to disappear without questions being asked, certainly not in early 1943 when there was no danger of their liberation by Allied forces, or of Japan being soundly defeated in battle.

Initial conditions in the new camp were, in the words of Major Hankins, 'very unsatisfactory due to low temperatures, inadequate housing and insufficient medical service.'[7] But as we shall discover, the conditions at Mukden were considerably better than those in almost every other Japanese prison camp that have been documented by historians, including myself, over the course of several books on this highly-emotive subject. The fact that the Japanese intended the present camp to be only a temporary prison was the main reason why the facilities were extremely basic and harsh at the beginning.

The camp consisted of an area enclosed by a double barbed-wire fence with crisscrossed sections in between the two fences that stood four feet apart, each fence standing only three-and-a-half feet high. The POW accommodation buildings comprised nineteen long, low, double-walled wooden barracks. Each barrack block was 125 feet long and fourteen feet wide and sunken two feet into the earth – as was the Chinese custom in this region – to provide some protection and insulation from the elements. The POWs were assigned in groups of between seventy to ninety men to each barrack block, where they would sleep on a raised wooden platform six feet wide and extending the length of each side of each half of the building. The middle of each building had a main entrance and two side doors at each end. The barrack floor was constructed out of cold hard brick and furniture was minimal; each hut assigned only two or three wooden tables and benches. The officers were housed separately from the men in their own barrack block which due to their lower numbers, was considerably less crowded.

Mitsubishi was 'so anxious to have as many prisoners as they could get to this large complex of factories that the first group of POWs who arrived ... found that no accommodation had been prepared for them,'[8] states historian Linda Goetz Holmes who wrote a damning indictment of Mitsubishi's use of Allied POWs as slave labour during the Second World War. 'When we got up in the morning, the frost on the bricks looked like it had snowed,' recalled former American POW Gene Wooten. The prisoners were forced to march five miles to work every day. Before production could begin at the factories, the prisoners had to construct the buildings themselves, a major civil engineering project that offered huge scope for sabotage. 'Every time we poured concrete, we buried as many tools as we could,' said Leo Padilla, one of the Americans who were forced to build the MKK machine tool factory. 'We must have buried a hundred shovels under that factory floor.'[9]

THE CAMP

One of the best ways in which to fully understand the Mukden Camp is to compare it with another camp, also in China, of a similar size that was also stocked primarily with American prisoners. Woosung Camp was located close to where the Huangpu River empties into the East China Sea, about fifteen miles from the centre of Shanghai. One of the few Britons imprisoned at Woosung was Sir Mark Young, the former Governor of Hong Kong, who was captured by the Japanese when the colony surrendered on Christmas Day 1941. After the war Young provided the British government with a detailed report about the camp. 'There were about 1,500 prisoners and conditions, particularly as regards sanitation, were most unsatisfactory,'[10] he recalled. The camp contained a large proportion of American servicemen, members of the 'North China Marines', a group detached to guard the consulate in Beijing and the consulates and concessions at Tientsin (now Tianjin) and Chinwangtao (Qinhuangdao), under the command of Colonel William W. Ashurst. In Shanghai, as elsewhere, the Japanese 'had deliberately chosen run-down and overgrown sites for the internees and did nothing to prepare the facilities for occupation in advance of the foreigners' arrival,'[11] commented Sir Mark. At Woosung, the wooden huts were originally constructed as a Chinese Nationalist barracks and in a bad state of repair. The camp covered about ten acres in area and was enclosed by an electrified fence. There were seven barracks, each building about seventy feet long and twenty-five feet wide. Next to the back door of each hut there was a squat toilet and wash rack. Inside each barrack block a long corridor ran down the centre with a series of rooms on each side that contained wooden sleeping bays. The Japanese crowded between two hundred and three hundred men into each barrack with eighteen or twenty to a room – considerably worse living conditions than those encountered at Mukden. On first sight the barracks painted a depressing picture. Window panes were missing here and there, the roofs leaked when it rained, parts of the floors were missing which meant prisoners had to be careful where they stepped, and because the walls had no insulation the men froze during the hard Shanghai winter.

Both Mukden and Woosung Camps had considerably better accommodations than those to be found along the Burma-Thailand Railway, a massive Japanese civil-engineering project that utilised Allied POWs and local peasants to construct a railway line through some of the toughest jungle on earth. Tens of thousands perished from disease, malnutrition, accidents and deliberate abuse by the guards. The buildings at Songkrei Camp could not have been more different from those provided to the prisoners at Mukden and Woosung. The barracks were constructed of bamboo with atap roofs but these were totally inadequate in the wet conditions of the jungle. Lieutenant-Colonel J.M. Williams of the Australian Pioneers, a senior Allied prisoner at several camps along the length of the railway, recalled: 'In one camp we spent five months in a very crowded area ... where for the first three weeks there was no roof on our building. I complained to the Japanese commander about the accommodation and he said that they were equally crowded. In fact, twenty-three officers and twenty-three other ranks of my Force occupied the same space as three Japanese soldiers.'[12] At Tan Toey Barracks Camp on Amboina in the Moluccas, 800 Australian and 300 Dutch POWs were imprisoned in February 1942. They had formed the pre-war garrison and had been captured after the fall of the Netherlands East Indies. Eight months after their arrival, 500 of the prisoners were moved to Hainan Island in southern China while the rest remained at Tan Toey until their liberation in September 1945. The Japanese progressively requisitioned the POWs accommodation blocks for their own use, including the creation of a bomb dump inside the camp perimeter that contained 200,000 pounds of high explosive and armour-piercing bombs. This massive pile of ordnance was just yards from the camp hospital and a separate compound that contained 250 Dutch women and children internees. Inevitably, Allied aircraft attacked the unmarked camp and its ammunition dump on 15 February 1943. 'Six Australian officers, four other ranks and twenty-seven Dutch women and children were killed, and twenty more Australian prisoners of war were badly wounded.'[13] Only 123 Australian POWs were still alive to be liberated in 1945.

Another camp typical of the appalling neglect of prisoner accommodation normally practised by the Japanese, was that on Haroekoe Island in the Moluccas. Two-thousand-and-seventy British and Dutch POWs were shipped to the small island in April 1943 to build an airstrip for the Japanese. The location of their camp was a strip of undrained swampy slope along the side of a hill. The accommodation consisted of a few huts built of bamboo,

The Camp

many minus sides and roofs. When the senior British officer, Squadron Leader Pitts of the RAF, complained, he was told that as prisoners they had no rights.

Turning back to Mukden Camp, fifty feet from the accommodation huts was the separate latrine block located inside a similar building to the barracks. Unlike at Woosung, the latrines were physically separated from the living quarters which was probably a healthier arrangement considering the level of sanitation inside the camp. There were twenty stalls and two long urinal troughs. The prisoners were not required to clean the latrines, except for mopping the floors, as the excrement was valuable and sold to local Manchurian peasants who used it to fertilise their fields. The so-called 'honey cart' was loaded up with the camp's combined excreta by Chinese and taken away – one of the few blessings that the prisoners could count upon. In other POW camps in other parts of Asia, prisoners were forced to ladle out the results of chronic diarrhoea and dysentery by hand, the Japanese guards delighting at their charges' disgust and shame with their humiliating task. As it was, going to the toilet at Mukden Camp could be a disgusting business, as imprisoned doctor Mark Herbst recalled: 'The latrines would frequently become so full in the winter that one would have to be careful how far down he squatted for fear of being met in the rear by a frozen pile of excreta extending up six or eight inches above and through the hole in the floor.'[14]

The toilet arrangements at Mukden were considerably superior to most found in Japanese POW camps. So too was the attitude to the spread of disease. At the Haroekoe Island Camp the Japanese constructed latrine trenches beside each bamboo hut. Dysentery outbreaks were extremely serious at this camp and the Japanese became so frustrated at the lack of fit men able to work that they called an officer's parade and beat all of the Allied officers present, including the senior British officer. So bad did the dysentery epidemic become at Haroekoe that there was a complete breakdown of medical facilities, such as they were. Dr. R. Springer, a Dutch Army Medical Corps doctor in the camp, recorded the grim results: 'Still diarrhoea cases in increasing numbers ... The sick are too weak to go to the lavatories, we have not enough tins and buckets inside the barracks for the purpose, so they go outside,

outside in the mud which is drenched with faeces and alive with maggots.'[15]

The Woosung Camp outside Shanghai stank, for the latrine facilities there were inadequate, and the squat toilets also had to be regularly emptied by Chinese coolies who used hand buckets. In the summer Sir Mark Young recalled that huge clouds of black flies swarmed around the latrines and invaded the rest of the camp, landing on the men's food and spreading dysentery bacteria. A plague of rats also infested the camp, constantly scampering under the huts and into the kitchen, their droppings adding to the collective filth.

Washing facilities at Mukden Camp consisted of a bathhouse with six large tanks located close to the latrine block. The prisoners were not allowed into the tanks. Instead, the warm water was dipped out with buckets to wash with. 'Due to the large numbers of men,' recalled Major Hankins, 'rosters were run on which a man got a bath once a week.'[16] The Japanese had actually two fully equipped bathhouses in the camp, but they only permitted one to operate.

The prisoners' food was prepared in the communal kitchen, with its attached dry storage room, icebox, and sleeping quarters for the Japanese mess sergeant who very strictly supervised the rations. The kitchen was actually under the day-to-day supervision of American Chief Warrant Officer A.A. Bochsel, with Sergeant Andrew Prevuznak as mess sergeant. The food issue remains contentious. According to some American veterans and historians, the prisoners were starved or certainly kept in a malnourished state. The American POWs arrived at the camp malnourished and suffering from vitamin deficiencies, but from the available evidence for some of the early months of imprisonment the food ration at Mukden was quite good, or certainly better than that received in other Japanese prison camps. This assertion is born out by the comments noted by Major Peaty in his secret diary. Perhaps, coincidentally, when prisoner death rates peaked in the early months of 1943, many witnesses reported medical examinations and regular inoculations which seems to run contrary to the expected trend if the Japanese were conducting no experimentation. 'There was never so much bitterness in this camp about distribution of food as there was in most other camps of which I have had reports,'[17] noted army doctor Captain Herbst. The daily

THE CAMP

average calorific intake of the prisoners at Mukden in early 1943 is perhaps the most obvious divergence from the usual Japanese prison camp pattern, indicating once again that something was quite different at Mukden as compared with almost anywhere else within the POW system. According to the British Department of Health Estimated Average Requirements (EAR) for 2011, the daily calories intake for men should be 2,550. Fortunately for us, Major Peaty kept a detailed diary where he often recorded the estimated daily calorific intake of the prisoners. Peaty was not a doctor, but there were other military doctors present among the officer prisoners who were well placed to judge calories, not to mention army medical orderlies and cooks. His entry for 5 April 1943 states: 'We estimate that we are receiving between 2,800 and 3,000 calories.' Ten days later on 15 April Peaty recorded: 'Calories now at about 2,200.' Again on 28 April Peaty wrote: 'Rations issued for the next three days give us about 2,000 calories.' The reports that were written by Major Hankins and US Army doctor Mark Herbst, detailed the prisoners receiving between 2,000 and 3,000 calories a day. Sometimes their calorific intake was slightly below that recommended by the British Government's current medical advisors, and sometimes above the average. Significant malnutrition cannot have been further exacerbated by a lack of calories in early 1943, and can probably be discounted as a factor in the large number of American deaths that occurred at Mukden during this time, pointing to some other explanation.

The bill of fare at Mukden consisted of a breakfast of bread and soup. Five ounces of bread were issued per man with a corned mush. For the first six months of the camp's operation each prisoner received about 200 grams of corn each day, though this was later reduced to 120 grams. There were three meals per diem, and fresh water was taken from wells and boiled before being drunk for safety reasons. The food was ladled into buckets in the kitchen and served to the men in their barrack blocks. Major Peaty repeatedly recorded in his diary that the Japanese gave the prisoners extra sources of food during 1943. On 10 May 'Fifteen ten-day old chicks arrived to start a poultry farm. They are believed to be Rhode Island Reds.' The following day's entry stated 'Rations have been slightly increased.' On 23 May Peaty wrote: 'Two eggs per man issued.'[18] The prisoners appear to have been receiving a better diet, according to Peaty, than in other camps studied by this author, as we shall see. A variety of food continued to be issued by the Japanese at Mukden, Peaty recording on 29 May 1943: 'Good potatoes (120kg) were issued to-day. Estimate 2,540 calories a day.'[19] In fact, the calories intake recorded on that date almost exactly matched what is now considered an average daily intake for modern men in Britain. '14 Jun 1943 – Rations have improved. We are now getting potatoes and fish in reasonable quantities, giving us about 3,000 calories.' Almost a month later and Peaty was completely satisfied with the rations, noting on 13 July: 'Food better than ever before: we are now getting cucumbers, and fish about twice a week.' 'Tomatoes issued – really excellent,'[20] Peaty penned just two days later.

At this point we must make a comparison between the rations and calories situation at Mukden and some other Japanese prisoner-of-war camps where figures have survived. The results are extremely revealing. At the aforementioned Tan Toey Barracks Camp on Amboina the food rations were 'adequate and reasonably good'[21] until July 1943. Thereafter, the prisoners were systematically starved. The ration scale fell rapidly, and when combined with hard labour that the prisoners were expected to undertake whether sick or fit, the death rates were appalling. A ration of just four ounces of rice and four ounces of sweet potatoes was issued daily to each prisoner. The Japanese guards, in comparison, received a daily allowance of fifteen ounces of rice that was supplemented by generous portions of fish and plenty of vegetables.

In North Borneo, the Japanese shipped in 1,496 Australian soldiers taken prisoner in Singapore in February 1942. They were housed at a frightful place named Eight Mile Camp and brutally treated. They were needed to construct an airfield for the Japanese. Conditions at the camp steadily deteriorated throughout 1943 and 1944. By the beginning of 1945 the daily ration for each prisoner had been reduced to a small quantity of tapioca and sweet potatoes, a few greens and one four ounce cup of rice per day, equating to less than 1,000 calories per man per day. Conditions inside the camps that sprouted up in the jungle along the route of the infamous Burma-Thailand 'Railway of Death' were even more pitiful. Gunner Russell Braddon of the Australian Artillery noted that the prisoners were so hungry that they '… ate anything which was not actually poisonous, even, in Thailand, the fungus of trees.'[22] At Batu Lintang Camp on Borneo, a joint prisoner-of-war and civilian

THE CAMP

internment centre, the basic diet distributed by the Japanese that was deemed by them suitable for all of the prisoners contained a daily allowance of just 1.5 ounces of protein, equating to only 1,600 calories. At practically every camp that I have surveyed, rations, and therefore calorific intake, steadily decreased as the war progressed. Malnutrition or diseases that attacked immune systems already seriously weakened by a lack of food caused the greatest majority of the deaths that occurred in the camps. For the vast majority of military prisoners-of-war survival became a numbers game – calorific intake and quantity of rations versus the remaining months of the war. This does not appear to have been the case at Mukden, flying in the face of historically accepted Japanese practices for the treatment of Allied prisoners-of-war. It beggars the question of why this was the case – why did the Japanese bother to feed the POWs at Mukden reasonably well when they failed to do so in the vast majority of their camps? It can have nothing to do with keeping their labour force healthy and functional, if that was the reason for the POWs presence at Mukden, for elsewhere Allied POWs were expected to undertake much harder labouring projects like constructing airfields and building railways, when kept in a deliberate state of starvation by their captors.

Even though apparently reasonably well fed, the American prisoners (but not the British, Australians or New Zealanders) died in large numbers throughout the early months of their imprisonment at Mukden. Major Peaty kept a careful note of the death rates. On 24 February 1943 he noted that a funeral service was held for the 186 Americans who had died in the past *105* days. Worse was to come. Peaty appeared to identify the cause of these deaths as he constantly makes references to rampant diarrhoea and dysentery affecting many of the prisoners in his secret and contemporary diary. It appears from Peaty's diary that the Japanese were not deliberately starving the prisoners, which normally caused malnourished prisoners to perish from treatable diseases like dysentery. These men were quite healthy and robust as compared with other prisoners held by the Japanese, yet their mortality rate was staggering, and as bad, or perhaps even worse, than camps with much more inferior facilities and food. The question is simple: what was killing them? Perhaps the most perplexing of all is the fact that not one British or

Australian prisoner who shared the same food, accommodation, work, recreation and latrines with the Americans, died. The law of averages suggests that some of them should have succumbed to the same disease as their American comrades, but none of them did. This fact simply does not make sense and is one of the biggest suggestions that the disease was not naturally occurring. It is either a very large coincidence or the Americans were getting ill through some artificial means, perhaps associated with the visit to the camp of Japanese medical personnel. We shall look into this fascinating anomaly in more detail later.

With so many men sick and dying, what were the medical facilities like at Mukden Camp? They were quite basic, though for such a small camp there was an over abundance of medical officers that was certainly unusual when compared with other Japanese POW camps in Asia. Aside from the POW doctors, most notably Captains Herbst and Brennan, there were at all times at least three Japanese Army doctors at the camp out of a total of four who had been assigned there. This fact does tend to lend some weight to the hypothesis that the Japanese were conducting experiments inside the camp, as it was extremely unusual, perhaps unique, to find a Japanese prison camp that was so well stocked with medical personnel. Under normal conditions prisoners were left to fend for themselves. Any perusal of the hundreds of histories of the camps along the Burma-Thailand Railway, or those in Japan or the Philippines, supports this historical view. For example, the rampant dysentery outbreak at the Haroekoe Island Camp was treated simply. The Japanese medical officer called a parade of all the British and Dutch officers on 21 June 1943. He told them that the dysentery was their own fault. 'All you have to do is to kill all the flies and cut your finger nails and the epidemic will die down.'[23] Perhaps it is not surprising that of the 2,070 British and Dutch POWs who were held in this camp, less than 50 per cent survived the war.

It is tempting to ascribe the presence of so many Japanese Army doctors at the Mukden Camp to supporting the work of Unit 731 scientists who appear to have visited the camp on several occasions. As we will shortly see, a Unit 731 scientist did later confirm that in 1942–43 he was stationed at the local Mukden Military Hospital along with other scientists who worked for Dr. Shiro Ishii, the

THE CAMP

creator of Unit 731, allowing them easy access to the prison camp just a few miles away.

Eventually, there were four wooden barrack blocks used exclusively as medical facilities by the Japanese at the Mukden Camp – a considerable amount of bed space for such a tiny camp. There was a main hospital building with a Japanese doctor's office, a sick call and treatment room, and a pharmacy. US Army doctor Captain Herbst stated in postwar testimony that most of the illnesses that he treated were for 'upper respiratory infections, dysentery and diarrhoea, and avitaminotic neuritis [caused by vitamin deficiencies in the POW diet?] mostly sensory.' He added that 'practically no medicine was available.'[24] What medicine there was had to be carefully rationed. Aspirin in crystal form was sparingly doled out. Sulfonamide was almost non-existent and it was only used on patients who were suffering from severe pneumonia. 'Morphine or opium for the dysenteries was not forthcoming from the Japs unless the doctors practically got on their knees to beg for it,'[25] recalled Herbst. Nutritional deficiencies in the diet were partly offset by prescribing three grams of brewer's yeast ingested three times weekly.

Herbst recalled that the Japanese medics lived at the east end of the so-called 'hospital.' The sick call room was later converted into offices. One of the hospital barracks was used as a dysentery ward and another building was utilised as an isolation unit for diphtheria cases. The barrack block behind was used for chest diseases, both acute and chronic. The difficulties that the POW doctors faced were numerous. 'Cooperation from the Japs was, at best, poor,' recalled Herbst. 'Language difficulties on diagnoses and medication were great.'[26] To ease some of the language and cultural misunderstandings, two of the enlisted prisoners who acted as medics learned almost fluent spoken, and workable written, Japanese.

Compared with other camps the medical facilities at Mukden appear to have been unusually extensive for such a small prisoner population. Major Cyril Wild, who spoke Japanese and had interpreted for Lieutenant General Arthur Percival when he had surrendered the Singapore garrison in February 1942, was held at Songkrei Camp on the Burma-Thailand railway construction project in August 1943. He testified at the Tokyo War Crimes Trial what he had witnessed concerning the 'medical facilities' that were available at his camp. Wild recalled that inside a hut lay 700 men arranged two deep along each side on shelves. All of them were painfully thin and nearly naked. Down the middle of the hut were around 250 men who were suffering from tropical ulcers. 'These commonly stripped the whole of the flesh from a man's leg from the knee to the ankle,' Wild stated. 'There was an almost overwhelming smell of putrefaction.'[27] Sickness was endemic among the prisoners. Cholera roared up and down the railway line, killing hundreds each time it struck, and the usual POW diseases of malaria, dysentery and typhus carried off many hundreds more. The Japanese did not appear to care one iota, and in fact, issued ridiculous rules that made the situation even worse. Major Wild related that only fifteen per cent of the prisoners were 'allowed' to be sick at any one time, and only permitted *one* disease at a time. Everyone else had to work – and work fast – on starvation rations. The choices forced upon prisoner doctors were terrible and not something the POW medics at Mukden ever encountered: 'One British doctor and his work detail officer had a private formula,' writes Gavan Daws in *Prisoners of the Japanese*. 'Take two men, one classified as sick, the other as sickest. Send the sick man out to work and he would probably die. Keep the sickest in camp and he would certainly die. But keep the man who was merely sick back in camp and he had a better chance of surviving. That was medical ethics under the Japanese.'[28] Each mile of track laid through the jungle eventually cost the lives of sixty-four Allied prisoners and 240 native workers. The sobriquet 'Railway of Death' was well earned in this case.

If the Burma/Thailand Railway is an extreme example of Japanese neglect of the health and welfare of prisoners-of-war, there are many other camps that provide an equally depressing story. At Batu Lintang Camp on Borneo, the resident Japanese medical officer, Lieutenant Yamamoto, created a camp hospital. Prisoners tried to avoid this building as much as possible for it was filthy and resembled a morgue rather than a treatment centre. Yamamoto, a doctor, actually violently beat any patients who had the temerity to ask for medicines, and indeed, was so slovenly and incompetent, that apart from issuing orders that stated sick prisoners would receive no rations, left the actual medical duties to the several doctors among the prisoners. Yamamoto's attitude to sick prisoners was summed up by one prisoner doctor as 'live and

The Camp

let die.' The prisoners clubbed together and tried to produce a stock of food and drugs with which to help those who were sick, but the death rate was such that special re-useable hinged coffins were used because of a shortage of wood. Burials occurred virtually every single day of the war. The death rate among the British POWs and male internees was appalling, with two thirds – equating to around six hundred – of these men dead by the time of liberation in September 1945. But tropical diseases and disorders stalked all of the prisoners, regardless of their gender or their age. Tropical ulcers would turn septic without treatment and kill; dysentery was rife due to the poor sanitation in the camp, and malaria, beri-beri, dengue fever, scabies, septic bites and sores killed hundreds of others. Neither of the examples discussed from Thailand and Borneo was particularly 'special' – pick up any book about the experiences of Allied POWs in Japanese hands and such stories are legion.

One story that perhaps explains the Japanese attitude to dysentery, and to prisoners' illnesses in general, comes from the Haroekoe Island Camp. When compared with the apparent concern that was demonstrated by Japanese physicians at Mukden Camp to the outbreak of dysentery among the prisoners, the British and Dutch POWs moved by hell ship to Haroekoe Island in April 1943 could not believe the cruelty of their Japanese captors. 'We still believed in humanity even from the Nips, but that proved to be silly,' wrote Dutch Army doctor Springer in November 1945 in an official report about the treatment of the men under his care. You should bear in mind that these prisoners were moved to a new location to work as slave labourers on an important military construction project. 'I get the impression that the Nips were out for wilful murder. When we told them our fear for the future regarding the danger of spreading an epidemic of dysentery, and that we expected many death cases, we often got the answer, "nice when dead".'[29]

Chapter 5

Forced Labour

It was a regular thing for men to be made to stand with arms outstretched holding a bowl of water, and to receive a clout from a 'kendo stick' or wooden sword, if they spilt any water.

Major Robert Peaty, Mukden Camp

If the story so far tells us anything, it is that the Mukden Camp was not an ordinary run-of-the-mill POW centre. The prisoners received better food than their colleagues imprisoned in Thailand, the Philippines, Borneo and elsewhere, and the medical facilities were extraordinarily extensive for such a small camp. Oddly, it was packed with doctors and hospital huts, but not stocked with any medicines. The anomalies continue to pile up the closer one looks at Mukden, and the picture that is emerging is of a camp that was somehow 'special'. The prisoners did suffer privations from a poor diet to hard labour and physical punishment that you or I would find very difficult, but when held in comparison with the hellholes that served as POW camps elsewhere in Occupied Asia, the Mukden Camp did not even register. This fact was openly admitted just after the war by the senior British officer, Major Peaty, once he had had the opportunity to speak with other officers who had been sent to slave on the Burma-Thailand Railway or to Japan and Korea.

Our survey of Mukden Camp throws up yet more strange facts on a closer inspection. The supply situation at the temporary camp at Mukden was relatively good compared with normal life under Japanese rule. Although only one change of Japanese winter clothing was issued to the prisoners on their arrival in November 1942, each man did receive six blankets, a pillowcase and sheets, and a straw mattress to sleep on. Compare this with Makassar Camp in the Netherland East Indies where the prisoners had no furniture, no bedding and no issue of clothing.

A donation of 1,500 yen from the Vatican in Rome was used to purchase athletic equipment, clocks, and musical instruments – practically unheard of luxuries within the Japanese prison camp system. At Makassar Camp the Japanese commandant, on pain of a severe beating, banned even singing. In addition, the Mukden Camp canteen had limited supplies of cigarettes, soybean sweets, combs, and hair pomade, all of which could be purchased using the pay the prisoners each received from the Japanese. Officer prisoners received the basic pay of Japanese officers of the same rank. Officers of field rank received 30 yen a month, and company officers 27 yen a month, but they were expected to reimburse the Japanese for the cost of their subsistence and clothing (effectively paying for the privilege of being prisoners). The other ranks received a basic allowance of 20–40 sen (100 sen = 1 yen) per day depending on how much work they performed in the local factories that were soon created close to the new camp.

Recreation was also possible, again an almost unheard of luxury in a Japanese POW camp. There was a recreation field where the Americans played softball. 'A few individually owned books were brought into the camp principally by the British prisoners and were given a limited circulation.'[1] An unproductive vegetable garden was begun outside of the wire. Although there were no chaplains among the POWs, the Japanese nonetheless permitted the officers to hold services, including burial services, an Easter and Christmas service, and also respected religious freedom. These kinds of activities were usually severely proscribed in most camps.

Contact with the outside world was, as in most Japanese prison camps, severely limited. In April, and again in July 1943, the prisoners were permitted to send one twenty-five-word postcard to relatives. The camp's outgoing post was limited to three letters and three postcards per annum for officers, and one letter and three postcards for the Other Ranks. This was again a luxury, whereas at the aforementioned Makassar Camp the prisoners received no mail whatsoever during their imprisonment and neither were they allowed to send any out. The Japanese heavily censored all outgoing mail from Mukden Camp and any mention of the conditions under which the prisoners were living and working would result in the communication being destroyed or the prisoner being punished. During the entire duration of their imprisonment at Mukden, none of the prisoners received any post from home – the Japanese routinely embargoed this. Nevertheless, the fact that the Japanese permitted the prisoners to send out post once again raises a red flag concerning the purpose of the camp. In other camps the Japanese occasionally forced prisoners to write extremely short postcards to their relatives stating that they were happy and being well treated by their captors, but this was simply a propaganda exercise by the Japanese.

Certainly, the prisoners at Mukden had very little idea of how the war was progressing, and it appears from the available evidence that none of the prisoners who were held at Mukden were caught with 'illegal' information and were punished. In other camps this was not the case. For example, at River Valley Road Camp 17 near Omuta in Japan, the commandant was informed that an American prisoner by the name of Hubbard had been caught with a scrap of a Japanese newspaper on his person. The Japanese, and especially the *Kempeitai* military police, were obsessed with preventing news of the disastrous progress of the war falling into prisoners' hands and they went to extraordinary lengths of barbarity to root out radio receivers and news sheets in the camps. Inevitably, Hubbard was beaten up by a group of camp guards and then thrown into the guardhouse. The commandant informed the local *Kempeitai*. 'Next day three Kempeitai corporals came to the camp. They beat Hubbard ... with their rifle butts. [For] Four days Hubbard's screams echoed across the subdued camp – until merciful death claimed him at last.'[2]

The prisoners at Mukden had no idea that they were often receiving considerably better treatment and enduring better conditions than their comrades in the Philippines, Borneo and Thailand. Only Major Robert Peaty, the senior British officer at Mukden, became aware that his men were better treated than the poor souls shipped out of Changi Camp in Singapore to a multitude of slave labour camps on the Railway of Death or in Korea and Japan. In December 1945, Peaty wrote a detailed report on the Mukden Camp for his superiors. Although he acknowledged that, in his opinion, and after consulting with fellow officers who had been

Forced Labour

imprisoned elsewhere in Asia, the Mukden Camp – both the temporary one and the later permanent one – was well-run and the men relatively well-treated, Peaty believed the reason for this unusual largesse from the Japanese was quite simple: 'Even while there, I formed the opinion that it was a 'propaganda' camp, for we received so many visits from the Japanese Propaganda Corps, who brought cine-cameras and took reels of baseball games, the men marching to work (with all Japanese guards well out of sight), quizzes, spelling-bees, camp orchestra and sing-songs at Christmas time, and so on ...'[3]

Peaty's assertion that Mukden was simply a 'propaganda' stunt is not entirely without some basis in fact. Senior Allied officers captured by the Japanese were held alongside Peaty's men, though separately, for a while before they were sent to separate camps as political prisoners. Their number included the former British commander of Malaya, Lieutenant-General Percival, the American commander in the Philippines, Lieutenant-General Jonathan Wainwright, and a large number of major generals, brigadiers and full colonels. Many bemoaned the constant filming they were subjected to by the Japanese. But it made sense to use the enemy's most senior officers as propaganda tools. What interest was there in a small camp of a few thousand ordinary enemy POWs? Perhaps the intermittent filming that Peaty refers to was actually for an entirely different purpose?

* * *

The Japanese guards who worked at Mukden Camp were seconded from regular units of the Kwantung Army stationed nearby, though the commandant and his staff officers were on permanent attachment. There is one aspect of the Mukden Camp that appears to be reasonably different from the general picture of Allied imprisonment by the Japanese. As noted by several of the senior Allied officers who were imprisoned inside the camp, the Japanese desisted in the main from torturing and abusing their charges to the degree recorded elsewhere in Asia. Senior American officer Major Stanley Hankins stated: 'There were one or two incidents when men were severely beaten and confined without trial.'[4] Hankins also recalled: 'There were no serious cases of mistreatment other than face slapping ...'[5] Major Peaty stated that none of the prisoners were arbitrarily killed by the guards, 'but two men

(Americans) who were badly beaten up, died about fourteen days later. As they were perfectly hale and hearty before being beaten up, and on coming out of the guard-house they just took to their beds and died, I believe that what they had endured was the primary cause of their deaths.'[6] In fact, the only deaths that can be directly attributed to Japanese brutality were the executions of three prisoners who had tried to escape just before the permanent camp was created four miles away from the temporary one in July 1943. A month before, on 21 June 1943, the three Americans, Sergeant Joseph B. Chastain and Corporal Victor Paliotti of the US Marine Corps, along with Seaman 1st Class Ferdinand Meringolo of the US Navy, had broken out of the temporary camp and fled into the countryside. Unfortunately for them, they were soon apprehended by Japanese patrols, proving that it was extremely difficult to remain on the run without assistance from locals when deep behind enemy lines. Any white face stood out among the Asian community and such was the level of terror that the Japanese managed to instill in local communities that few civilians, even though they would have sympathised with the men's plight, would have risked the awful retribution of the *Kempeitai* had they been caught. 'On 7 Jul 43 at least seven men were severely beaten by 1st Lt. Miki (Superintendent Officer), and later confined without food,' recalled Hankins, as the Japanese investigated further into the behaviour of the prisoners. These prisoners were deemed to have colluded with the escaped men and were brutally punished. Major Hankins added: 'The group remained in the Guardhouse until the latter part of October '43. The three men who escaped were captured on or about 2 July, tried by military court and executed at 5:20 o'clock, 31 July '43. We were informed unofficially that reason for the death penalty was due to the death of one Manchurian police and the wounding of another at the time of their recapture.'[7]

The executions of the three escapees appears to have been the only deaths that have been directly attributed to the Japanese camp staff, which was in itself unusual when compared with most other POW camps, as will be shown shortly.

Major Peaty made a careful study of some of the Japanese methods used to punish and humiliate prisoners at Mukden – and in this regard we find a fairly large amount of evidence that the non-terminal punishment methods employed by the Japanese at

Forced Labour

Mukden were similar to camps all across Asia. 'It was a regular thing for men to be made to stand with arms outstretched holding a bowl of water,' recalled Peaty, 'and to receive a clout from a "kendo stick" or wooden sword, if they spilt any water.' Peaty recounted another method of punishment employed by the guards. 'Men were also made to hold their arms above their heads and at the same time adopt a "knees bend" position. Again, as soon as the muscles tired and the position could no longer be held, a whack across the back of the legs was handed out.'[8] However, it appears that the Mukden POWs were spared a regime that was deliberately designed to trick prisoners into making mistakes so that they could be punished. Before Generals Percival, Wainwright, and cohorts were shipped to a camp in Manchuria, they were held on the island of Formosa. At Kwarenko Camp the senior British, American and Dutch officers and colonial officials were terrorised. Severe beatings were handed out for the most trivial of offences. For example, General Percival was beaten up for having a speck of dirt under one of his fingernails. The Japanese reason for this outrageous behaviour was their belief that by enforcing such regulations the spread of disease would be controlled. They did absolutely nothing to improve hygiene conditions inside the camp. Another camp rule stated that all prisoners, regardless of rank, had to have every clothing button fastened at all times, even when asleep. Japanese guards would often burst into the Generals' sleeping quarters in the middle of the night to conduct an 'inspection' and anyone failing this was beaten up. Throughout the Japanese prison camp empire, POWs, regardless of their rank, were forced to salute any Japanese soldier they encountered and to bow deeply to him. Thus, a British lieutenant general was expected to salute and bow to a Japanese private. Failure to do so resulted in a face-slap or worse. Any complaints that were made by senior Allied POWs to the camp commandant resulted merely in more punishments.

Although the POWs at Mukden were often struck or kicked by Japanese guards, and harsh though this 'corporal punishment' may appear to us now, it was tame when compared with many of the other Japanese camps, and the personality of the commandant appears to have played a major role in determining how unpleasant life was made for the inmates. Captain Susumu Hoshijima, commandant of the three prisoner-of-war camps set up at Sandakan in

Borneo, forbade prisoners inside the different camps from communicating with each other. Any resistance to this order, however minor, was met with a series of severe and increasingly mediaeval punishments. Inventive in his tortures, Hoshijima had ordered the construction of an instrument of pain that was quickly labelled 'The Cage' by the Australian and British POWs who suffered within it. It was located next to a big tree in Camp 1 and consisted of a wooden structure 130cm high and 170cm long, with iron bars on all sides. The Japanese ordered prisoners under punishment to sit at attention inside this cage for hours on end. The guards took a perverse delight in torturing the prisoners still further during their already intolerable confinement. Nineteen-year-old Private Keith Botterill, an Australian POW, recalled years later his experience inside the cage: 'The time I was in for forty days there were seventeen of us in there. No water for first three days. On the third night they'd force you to drink till you were sick. For the first seven days you got no food. On the seventh day they started feeding you half camp rations ... Every evening we would get a bashing, which they used to call physical exercise ...'[9]

At Makassar Camp, prisoners under punishment were forced to climb trees that were full of red ants and remain there. 'They were beaten into unconsciousness resulting in bruises and cracked ribs. The commandant himself took part in the beatings.'[10] Some of the beatings administered at Makassar were monumental. For example, 'On 4th August 1944 one English prisoner was given seventy strokes by Yoshida [camp commandant] personally because he had not given "eyes right" to the commandant's satisfaction.'[11] On another occasion, a stoker of the Royal Navy named Wilkinson, 'failed to obey some order which resulted in a working party leaving camp short of one man. Yoshida decided that Wilkinson should receive a beating. The stoker's endurance maddened the commandant, and Wilkinson had been given more than two hundred strokes before the punishment ended.'[12] Wilkinson was then forced to stand to attention for a further two hours.

Between May and August 1943, the prisoners labouring to construct the Burma-Thailand Railway through largely virgin jungle were subjected to the Japanese 'Speedo' campaign in which local commanders were ordered to speed up the construction to meet totally unrealistic deadlines created by army headquarters.

Forced Labour

Their Japanese, Korean and Formosan guards hounded the Allied prisoners and native workers relentlessly. The resulting mountain of corpses numbered several thousand. The guards became crazed, constantly screaming 'Speedo!' as they bashed prisoners in a lather of impotent rage, trying to fulfill their illogical and unrealistic orders with the same bloody-minded obedience with which Japanese soldiers launched mass charges into the teeth of Allied machine gun fire on the battlefield. The guards 'belted the men hourly with bamboos and rifle butts, or they kicked them,' recalled one Australian senior officer prisoner, Lieutenant-Colonel Williams. 'I have seen them use a five pound hammer and anything they could lay their hands on. One man had his jaw broken with a blow from a rifle butt because he bent a spike while driving it into the rail.'[13]

At Woosung Camp outside of Shanghai in China, in a camp that bore some similarities to Mukden in its appearance and in the size of its prisoner population, one of the Japanese Army interpreters preyed upon the inmates relentlessly. Army interpreters often wielded power well beyond their official position, and many absolutely loathed white men, often this animosity being derived from their experiences of living or studying in Western countries. Isamu Ishihara was technically a civilian, as were all interpreters in the Imperial Army, but like many other linguists he dressed like an officer (minus badges of rank), wore a holstered automatic pistol and carried a *samurai* sword. He was an extremely self-important and proud man, but on his arrival at the Shanghai camp he had been instructed by the real officers to salute the enlisted Japanese guards, which had caused him to loose a tremendous amount of face, hierarchies being extremely important to the Japanese. Ishihara used to take out his concomitant fury on the mostly American prisoners. 'He would beat POW officers with the sword till he was frothing, tell them they should kill themselves for being prisoners, and offer them his sword to do it. No one took him up.'[14] Sir Mark Young, the British Governor of Hong Kong who was briefly imprisoned at the camp, was spared any physical run-ins with this particular interpreter, except on one occasion when Sir Mark refused to salute him and Ishihara drew his sword and threatened then and there to cut the Governor's head off. Ishihara was nicknamed 'The Beast of the East' by the US Marine Corps prisoners at Woosung, and the name was appropriate. 'He used to say that when Japan won the war he was going to take a shit on the Stars and Stripes.'[15] His spoken English was not as good as he believed, and when he became excited or angry, which was pretty often, he tended to mangle his pronunciation or use the wrong words, particularly over the obsessive issue of saluting. 'If a prisoner did not salute him he would scream, "Why you not giving me SOLUTION?"'[16]

The description of Interpreter Ishihara is perhaps a little comic, but the reality of the man was far from humorous, particularly for those on the receiving end of his impotent rage. He was extremely violent, so much so that the Japanese camp commandant eventually took his sword away from him because he was constantly beating the prisoners with it or threatening to decapitate them (in its place he began carrying a riding crop with a heavy wooden handle which he employed equally liberally against all those who displeased him in some way). His other tortures were macabre and extremely sadistic, his favourite being a variation on the water torture that was used extensively by the Japanese throughout their prison camp system. The Ishihara version, used to extract 'the truth' from prisoners, involved the following: 'Prop a ladder on a slope, tie the prisoner to it, feet higher than head, pound something into his nostrils to break the bones so he had to breathe through his mouth, pour water into his mouth till he filled up and choked, and then it was talk or suffocate.'[17] Ishihara's other favoured torture was called the 'Finger Wire'. 'This involved using a contraption that bent a prisoner's finger back until it broke or was dislocated.'[18]

The physical abuses that the prisoners suffered at Mukden may have been much less invasive and permanently damaging than the tortures that were practised in camps such as Woosung, but they were nonetheless contraventions of the accepted Rules of War as laid down in agreements at The Hague and Geneva. Major Peaty's view was that the 'torture' methods that he witnessed being used 'were mostly brought into use when men had been caught out breaking camp rules, and were adopted in lieu of putting a man in detention on bread and water and without bedding.' Peaty stated that in his opinion associating the word 'torture' with these unusual Japanese disciplinary procedures was not entirely accurate. 'It does not compare with bamboo splinters under the nails, and so on, which I have heard of having happened at other camps.'[19] But at Mukden there was a great deal of minor incidences of violence that were perpetrated by the guards against their charges. 'Beatings were of such frequent occurrence that one ceased to take note of them as being anything out of the ordinary run,'[20] wrote Peaty in 1945, a comment that tends to corroborate Major Hankins' previous comments on this subject.

Japanese soldiers were so ready to resort to physical violence when enforcing their military codes of behaviour on POWs largely because they thought a slap in the face, or a kick, was perfectly normal. During their own initial recruit training, the instructors had constantly beaten the recruits until the young soldiers believed that once one was in a position of authority, lashing out to maintain that authority was legal and right. Of course, this was complete anathema to the military ethos of the British and United States armies, where it was considered a serious offence if an officer or NCO struck one of his soldiers. So it is perhaps understandable that largely ill-educated peasant soldiers from Japan, Korea and Formosa, might behave with such casual brutality towards the POWs in their care. The term 'face-slapping' does not do justice to the bashings that the prisoners received. Many officers and men have recounted that one was normally struck hard enough across the face to leave a bruise. Japanese guards also regularly used whatever they may have had in their hands at the time, from a rifle butt in the face, to a bamboo cane across the back, or a sheathed sword to the head and shoulders. Some guards enjoyed inflicting pain on POWs for a variety of psychological reasons and some only did the minimum that was required of them. A few even secretly helped the POWs to survive by slipping them food or excusing them duties. But the strong institutional focus of the Imperial Army, coupled with the Confucian concepts of loyalty and an obsession with 'face' and hierarchy, did combine to produce sometimes astounding acts of cruelty and sadism, as the few examples recounted earlier have graphically demonstrated.

* * *

In July 1943 the entire camp at Mukden was closed and all prisoners were marched under guard to a new camp located very close to the Mukden city limits. The apparent reason for this sudden change was so that the Japanese could employ the prisoners more effectively as labourers inside a series of Mitsubishi-owned factories they had set up close by Mukden in late 1942. This was a breach of the Geneva Convention, for prisoners may not be used to aid an enemy's military economy. The orders had come direct from the Japanese Prime Minister, General Hideki Tojo, in his dual capacity as Minister of War. Tojo had written instructions to camp commandants that explicitly stated: '... you must not allow them [prisoners-of-war] to lie idle, doing nothing but enjoy free meals, for even a single day. Their labour and technical skill should be fully utilized for the replenishment of production, and contribution thereby made toward the prosecution of the Greater East Asiatic War for which no effort ought to be spared.'[21]

In the case of the Mukden Camp, once again the prisoners received a much fairer treatment than that handed out to most other prisoners who laboured for the Japanese. For one thing, they were paid wages by the Japanese, and therefore were not technically slave labourers, unlike their unfortunate comrades who slaved and died building the Burma-Thailand Railway, or perished carving out airstrips on jungle-covered Pacific islands, or were sent down the mines in Japan and Korea. The camp also received a new name once the transfer was completed, becoming 'Hoten Camp No. 1'. In the summer of 1944 the Japanese set up a series of branch camps where work groups of prisoners and guards laboured in the various local Japanese concerns alongside Chinese labour. Branch No. 1 was at a tannery owned and operated by Manshu Leather, and the 150 Allied prisoners employed there formed Work Group C. Branch No. 2 employed a further 150 men (Work Group E) to work in a textile factory owned by Manshu Machinery Manufacturing Company. Work Group F numbered 125 men at Branch No. 3 who laboured inside a combination steel and lumber mill. A separate camp known as Branch CT was established 150 miles north and was used to imprison the aforementioned senior American, British, Australian and Dutch officers – mainly brigade commanders, staff colonels, military aides and batmen. This camp numbered 316 all ranks. The last camp was Sian Camp, a branch of the Hoten Camp that was established ten miles further north of Branch CT in December 1944, and which held only thirty-three of the very highest-ranking Allied officers and diplomats who had been captured by the Japanese, including the last commander of the Philippines, Lieutenant General Wainwright, the Governor of Malaya, Sir Shenton Thomas, and the defeated British commander in Malaya and Singapore, Lieutenant General Percival.

Conditions inside Hoten Camp No. 1 (which will continue to be described as 'Mukden Camp') were better than those already described at the temporary camp. The men received better rations, more comfortable living quarters and increased 'luxuries', such as cigarettes, sweets and recreational equipment. For those men who were transferred out to the working groups, although their branch camps were located close to Mukden City, the conditions were harder. The Japanese sent no officers with them, which meant they found it difficult to represent themselves to the Japanese, who being extremely hierarchical, did not entertain the opinions of the other ranks (for that matter the opinions of Allied officers were more often than not ignored as well).

On 24 May 1944 a group of 150 prisoners from Mukden Camp was transferred by ship to Kamisha, Japan, where the industrial giant Mitsubishi owned and operated a mine requiring slave labourers. In June 1944, a further fifty prisoners, all Americans, were sent to Kamisha as a punishment for acts of sabotage that they had committed while working in the factories at Mukden. As we saw earlier, during the construction of the factories the prisoners had buried shovels in the concrete floors. Once the factories were operational they had become more inventive in their sabotage techniques. Machinery was tampered with and many of the products made were defective. Industrial sabotage represented one of the only ways that prisoners of the Japanese could strike back at their captors – and it was widely practised by Allied working parties throughout Asia. The punishments for being caught were usually terrible, ranging from a death sentence to imprisonment or, as in the case at Mukden, transshipment to a far harsher working environment where many later perished.

Chapter 6

Guinea Pigs

As I can recall, it was in the beginning of 1943. At that time I was in a hospital in Mukden and research fellow Minata came to see me. He told me about his work and informed me that at the moment he was in Mukden to study [the] issue of immunity of American prisoners of war.

Major Tomio Karasawa, Section Head, Unit 731

A long line of thin white men stood patiently waiting to enter the hospital block. All of them were naked. Many of them joked among themselves, for it seemed that the Japanese were conducting another one of their regular medical inspections. Many grimaced at the thought of being prodded and poked by Japanese doctors for the umpteenth time but they had no choice. The white-coated doctors sat behind tables, while other assistants prepared hypodermic needles for the injections the Japanese were so fond of giving at the camp. The grumbling, joking and low murmur of conversation continued as the prisoners shuffled forward and was occasionally interspersed with some genuine levity when a prisoner revealed the ridiculous answers that he had created when questioned by the Japanese doctors – one Briton describing his pre-war occupation as 'race-horse urger'. But lurking around the edges of the queue were armed Japanese sentries, many holding sticks and other implements, occasionally shouting some command in a guttural and loud manner. The whole set-up was a little surreal, a fact not lost on many of the men taking part.

Guinea Pigs

Trying to fool the Japanese was apparently quite a keen sport among the prisoners at Mukden and it helped to relieve some of the tension. Peaty recorded: 'Many were the consultations that went on to think up more and more ridiculous things. One of them got a lot of fun out of classifying himself as a beer-taster, and another stated that his job was counting and checking "hundreds and thousands". They also looked up crazy things in the dictionary for hobbies, and all the "ologies" were shared round fairly equally. Philately, numismatics, bachanology, conchology, entomology (and etymology) were all among the things the lads were experts at.'[1]

There is not a single document proving beyond doubt that some of the Allied POWs held at Mukden Camp were the victims of nefarious medical experiments conducted by Japanese doctors from Unit 731. Instead, there exists a collection of many different sources from many different people giving places and times which, when taken collectively appear to suggest that human experimentation was performed at the Mukden Camp, and that Allied POWs were victims of that secret programme. To completely dismiss the body of evidence out-of-hand would be historically irresponsible and extremely shortsighted. Some historians who have written about Mukden Camp, including Linda Goetz Holmes, support the idea of Unit 731 involvement while others, like Sheldon H. Harris, have rejected the idea. The evidence remains debatable and contested in many quarters, not least by some of the men who survived their imprisonment in the camp, but when taken together many of the statements and documents corroborate each other, and many of the witnesses are impressive. One of the major issues which needs to be determined when dealing with such historically sensitive events is whether there was a cover-up after the war preventing the full truth of what occurred at Mukden from emerging. There is certainly a strong suggestion that this was the case.

Earlier, it was established from the reports and diaries of American and British officers who were held prisoner at the camp, that the POWs were receiving a daily calorific intake not far short of what is considered healthy and average for modern Britons. Although the American prisoners in particular arrived at Mukden from the Philippines in a poor state of health after their earlier experiences of Japanese captivity, it seems fair to suggest that none of the prisoners at Mukden Camp subsequently died from malnutrition or starvation. Major Peaty's detailed diary only talks about a dysentery-like illness carrying men off. The diet the prisoners received, according to the diaries of Peaty and Private Schreiner, later deteriorated considerably during 1944 and 1945, though in comparison with other prison camps the POWs were not too badly off. The POWs were also relatively humanely treated by their Japanese guards who appear, from the available evidence, to have refrained from torturing or arbitrarily murdering their prisoners, as was the case in many of the other camps that have been well-documented and studied across Asia. The reports of the American and British senior officers who were present at Mukden lists less than half-a-dozen men whose deaths were directly attributable to the Japanese administration, including three Americans who were shot for the crime of attempting to escape.

If the standard of subsistence in Mukden Camp was a little better than so many other comparable Japanese POW centres, and the administration slightly more benign, how was it that hundreds of American prisoners perished between arrival at the camp in late 1942 and the end of the war? What killed these men, and why were Americans the only ones who died? These deaths can be attributed to an outside intervention in the camp, from the introduction of a disease to selected members of the prisoner population, and, in other words, to the creation of an experiment.

Keeping the prisoners in relatively good health – as evidenced by the much better diet and increased calorific intake that has previously been noted in examinations of Mukden Camp – made admirable sense if it was the intention of the Japanese to use the prisoners as test subjects. We know that at the Pingfan facility the unfortunate Chinese, Manchurian and White Russian human guinea pigs that were held in the camp prison were well fed and kept disease-free so that when they were deliberately infected by doctors the test results were not interfered with by secondary infections and parasites. It also simply does not add up that so many Americans died, but not a single British, Australian or New Zealand prisoner, when all three groups shared the same food, sleeping quarters, washing facilities and latrines at Mukden Camp. The peculiar numbers of prisoners raises other questions; for example, why did the British and Commonwealth contingent together number approximately ten per cent of the total prisoner population? Why did the Japanese go to so much trouble to ship just 100 British and Commonwealth POWs all the way from Singapore to Mukden when they could just have easily added another 100 Americans to the transport that left the Philippines? The Mukden Camp seems to generate more questions than answers, but when taken together the rational explanations for these questions only strengthen the hypothesis that Allied prisoners held at that place were subject to Japanese human experiments, and the personnel who conducted them were part of Unit 731.

Unit 731 already had a history of using Caucasian prisoners in medical experiments. The practice had been going on for many years *before* the outbreak of the Pacific War in December 1941, and has been documented by Unit 731 veterans themselves who have bravely spoken out about what they did and saw. This fact alone should lead us to question the official American and British government denials that any Allied POWs were also used in this manner. Such a blanket denial flies in the face of common sense, especially after hundreds of thousands of Allied soldiers and civilians fell into Japanese hands after the great defeats that occurred in the face of the Japanese *blitzkrieg* across Asia of early 1942, providing a pool of human material that could have proven extremely useful to Shiro Ishii and his cohorts.

A former Japanese Youth Corps member who worked at Unit 731 from 1939 onwards and who spoke anonymously before an audience in Morioka City, Japan, in July 1994, stated: 'On many occasions, I saw prisoners taken from their cells wearing leg irons and made to move around the grounds. I think it was around spring of 1939 that I saw three mothers with their children in a test. One was a Chinese woman holding an infant, one was a White Russian woman with a daughter of four or five years of age, and the last was a White Russian woman with a boy of about six or seven.'[2] The witness related that they all perished as part of a low-level drop of typhoid or cholera bacteria from an aircraft.

Another anonymous Japanese witness who, as an army major had worked at Pingfan as a pharmacist, recounted his experiences to the Japanese newspaper *Mainichi* in November 1981. 'One time, I saw a technician at Unit 731, a field-grade officer, carrying out tests aimed at combating frostbite. Five White Russian women were used in the test at the time.'[3] One aspect of Unit 731 research that was taken very seriously was frostbite research and, in fact, it is the one area of research that has subsequently been acknowledged to have genuinely enhanced human understanding, though at the cost of an enormous amount of suffering and death. 'The technician placed the women's hands into a freezing apparatus and lowered its temperature to minus ten degrees Celsius, then slowly reduced the temperature to minus seventy degrees,' recalled the Japanese major. 'The condition of the frostbite was then studied. The result of the test was that the flesh fell from the women's hands, and the bones were exposed. One of the women had given birth in prison, and the baby was also used in a frostbite test. A little later, I went to look into the women's cells and they were all empty. I assume that they died.'[4]

From Japanese sources, it is clear that Unit 731 scientists had some interest in Caucasians. Turning now to what actually occurred at Mukden Camp – particularly during 1942–43 when witnesses recorded the most medical activity and deaths – it is clear that something out-of-the-ordinary took place. Major Peaty, as the senior British officer in the camp, carefully noted in his diary each visit by Japanese medical personnel, each inoculation that he and his men received, and the dates and numbers of deaths that occurred among the American prisoners. He never suggested where the illness that was killing the men originated, only that its symptoms were similar to dysentery and he appears to have believed that the Japanese were actually trying to help the prisoners by trying to eradicate it. Of course, Peaty had no idea at the time that the Japanese Army's concern for the health and wellbeing of the prisoners at Mukden was extremely unusual when placed into the context of the other camps, as we have seen previously. He also had no inkling, in common with all of the POWs and indeed their governments, that the Japanese were engaged in very large-scale human experimentation just a few hundreds miles away to the north in a secret and enormously well-funded operation employing thousands of scientists, researchers, technicians and soldiers.

The Japanese medical team visits were noteworthy to Peaty and have struck some historians of Japanese POW camps as virtually unprecedented in both the numbers of personnel sent and the frequency of the visits. According to Major Peaty, on 25 January 1943 '... there was an inspection by a General of the Japanese Medical Corps.' Two days later Peaty noted 'Inspection in quarters by two Japanese generals.' The very senior rank of the Japanese officers who came to the small camp does suggest a question: Why would they be interested in an insignificant camp with a small population of worthless white prisoners-of-war? It is especially pertinent to note that the inspections were made by generals from the Medical Corps, and not perhaps by curious field officers from local Kwantung Army units.

Major Peaty records that three days after the last inspection by the generals, 'Everyone received a 5cc Typhoid-para-typhoid A inoculation.'[5] This was what the prisoners were told they were receiving; they had absolutely no way of confirming that this Japanese statement was correct. On 5 February 1943 the prisoners were given a day off from working in the factory because it was Chinese New Year, and Peaty notes that the 'Japanese made use of the break to give everyone their second TAB [Typhoid injection].' Eight days later, on 13 February, Mukden Camp was visited again, this time by 'About 10 Japanese medical officers, and 20 other ranks ...' The medical personnel, who arrived in numbers never recorded before or after by historians in other Japanese POW camps, '... arrived to-day to investigate the cause of the large number of deaths,'[6] stated Peaty, who had presumably asked the Japanese commandant or his second-in-command for a clarification as was his right and duty as senior British officer. Major Stanley Hankins, the senior American officer in the camp, may also have informed him. On the following day, 14 February, Peaty wrote: 'Vaccination for small-pox.'[7] All the while these visits and inoculations were occurring, the deaths of American prisoners litter the pages of Peaty's diary. The numbers make sober reading, and a short summary drawn from Peaty's diary over just a few days works out thus: 20 January – two dead; 21 January – two dead; 22 January – one dead; 23 January – two dead; 24 January – one dead; 27 January – one dead; 29 January – two dead; 31 January – one dead; 4 February – two dead; 5 February – two dead; 9 February – one dead; 10 February – one dead. After a short lull, and following the 14 February 'Vaccination for small-pox' the deaths continued with two more Americans dying in hospital on the 15th and one on the following day.

The death rate appeared to spike not only around the time of the inoculations that Peaty recorded the prisoners as receiving, but also when fruit was suddenly, and uncharacteristically, distributed by the Japanese camp administration. On 25 January 'Forty cases of fresh fruit were received as a result of yesterday's inspection,' wrote Peaty. This fruit was distributed to the hospital patients, who continued to die at an alarming rate. On 29 January the Japanese issued more fruit. 'I believe it was one Chinese orange each – rather like a tangerine.'[8] Some American veterans later suggested that the Japanese had in some way doctored this fruit, as we will see.

On 15 February 1943 the Japanese medical team began examining the corpses of American prisoners who had died from the severe 'dysentery' which appeared to be doing the rounds of the camp. Peaty noted 'autopsies being performed on the corpses by the visiting Japanese.'[9] Private Sigmund Schreiner, an American prisoner, also recorded the autopsies in his secret diary: 'They [the Japanese] are going to perform autopsies on all the dead men in the warehouse. They look young to me, probably interns from the Mukden hospital.'[10] The autopsies were performed outside in the dead of winter. Shortly after these gruesome examinations were completed, and tissue and organ samples placed into glass jars and carefully labelled, another visit was made to the camp by a Japanese general. '18 Feb 1943. The Medical investigation is still in progress,' noted Peaty. 'Inspection by a Lieut-Gen. of the Japanese Medical Corps. Many high ranking officers have inspected us since our arrival. The purpose of their visits seems, as a rule, to be mere curiosity, for we do not observe that anything happens as a result of their inspections, except in the one case of the fruit which has already been noted.' Peaty records that the Japanese medical team questioned several of the Allied officers '... about dysentry [sic] and diarrhoea.' The only Japanese Medical Corps lieutenant generals who were permanently stationed in Manchuria at this time were Shiro Ishii of Unit 731 and Ryuji Kajitsuka, Chief of the Medical Section of the Kwantung Army (and Ishii's superior in the chain of command). This assumes that Peaty and the other officers were cogent with Japanese officer rank insignia, which it would be reasonable to assume that they were.

On 20 February 1943 all factory work was once more suspended by order of the Japanese and '... everyone was tested to find carriers and sufferers of dysentry and diarrhoea.'[11] The deaths among the American prisoners continued virtually on a daily basis: 19 February – one; 21 February – one. On 23rd Peaty attended a

Guinea Pigs

funeral service for 142 dead. In total, he noted, '186 have died in 105 days, all Americans.'

The findings of the medical investigation that Peaty supposed the Japanese had undertaken, generate more questions than they do answers. On 24 February Peaty secretly recorded, quoting the official Japanese explanation: 'The findings are "that ordinary diarrhoea, not usually fatal plus malnutrition and poor sanitation, and insufficient medicine, have proved a fatal combination of circumstances."'[12] Dealing with each part of the Japanese findings in turn, things do not quite add-up. Firstly, the cause of the 'ordinary diarrhoea' alluded to in the Japanese statement is not established. 'Malnutrition' could have been a major contributory cause, but the food had been improving since the arrival of the prisoners at the camp, and Major Peaty's diary entries confirmed that the prisoners were receiving between 2,200 and 3,000 calories each day, which is considered healthy today. Although some of the American POWs arrived at the camp in a malnourished state, they would probably have benefitted from the improved diet at the camp, rather than the reverse. At the very time that the Japanese conducted their medical investigation, Peaty was also moved to note in his diary that the men were receiving potatoes and fresh fish regularly, on top of their regular rations. On the question of 'poor sanitation, and insufficient medicine', these points ring true, based upon what we know of conditions inside the camp from the reports of Major's Hankins and Peaty, as well as US Army doctor Captain Mark Herbst. But this does not explain why only American POWs continued to sicken and die, and why British and Commonwealth prisoners living, eating and using the latrines alongside of them did not. The Japanese statement even admitted that 'ordinary diarrhoea' would not normally kill the afflicted.

We can establish that the prisoners should not have been terminally malnourished (that is suffering from starvation), if we accept the calorific intake figures recorded by Major Peaty, and it does not follow that the 'diarrhoea' would have been responsible for killing multiple numbers of one particular nationality. This would be the first disorder in medical history that was able to neatly differentiate between Americans, Britons, Australians, New Zealanders and Dutch (of which there was a handful in the camp). Something else, not identified in the Japanese statement, had to be the culprit behind the deaths. Whatever it was, the death toll was appalling. On 26 February two Americans died. The following day so did another. On 3 March 1943 Peaty recorded one American dead in the hospital, the next day two, and on the day after that, one more.

On 7 March 1943 the Japanese decided to quarantine the affected prisoners in one of the hospital wards, '... bringing the number of inmates up to 180.'[13] The deaths continued unabated, with another American serviceman succumbing to the mystery illness on 8 March. By 12 March Peaty was noting in his diary: '195 dead in 126 days.' Certain ill prisoners were even removed from the camp altogether and were sent to the Mukden Military Hospital. Interestingly, it came to light after the war that Unit 731 researchers conducted experiments inside the Mukden Military Hospital. Major Peaty noted that on 11 March 'Lt. Weeks (USA) was taken ... The patients [at the hospital] appear to be receiving good treatment in a ward set apart for Prisoners-of-War.' The deaths for the remainder of March make sobering reading: 16 March – one dead; 20 March – one dead in Mukden Military Hospital; 22 March – another death in Mukden Military Hospital; 23 March – two dead. Whilst all this was going on working parties of prisoners were outside of the camp working in the MKK factories where Peaty noted that their 'treatment is fairly satisfactory.'

On 19 April, with the winter nearly over and Peaty noting that 'The willow trees are beginning to show signs of greenness,' another large group of Japanese medics arrived at the camp to begin another 'investigation', 'as apparently the findings of the first one did not meet with approval.'

In May, the Japanese issued lime for use in the latrines, apparently in an effort to quell the breeding of disease-carrying flies, but on 24 May Peaty noted gravely in his diary 'Diarrhoea increasing.'[14] In the meantime more Americans had died in the camp or at the Mukden Military Hospital. By the end of May the camp cemetery contained 200 graves. At no time did the Japanese issue medicine to try and stem the tidal wave of diarrhoea and dysentery that tore through the camp, and which appears to have been an own goal for the Japanese. If they were serious about curing the ailments that were killing off large numbers of their factory workers, why did the Japanese not issue medicine at this time and end the men's suffering once and for good? They certainly possessed such medicines in their own base hospitals. The only conclusion that can be drawn from this strange state of affairs is that the Japanese medical investigation teams who toured the camp were not seeking a cure for the diarrhoea and dysentery problems, but rather that they were *observing* the effects of the diarrhoea and dysentery that they had artificially given to the prisoners as part of a test or experiment.

Major Peaty noted the apparent callousness of the Japanese medics towards the prisoners on 25 May 1943. 'While awaiting medicine for diarrhoea, (which was not forthcoming), men were ordered to exercise by playing baseball. The ball could not be found.' The following day the Japanese ordered a humiliating parade. 'Diagnosis of diarrhoea consists of running the men around the parade-ground, (I saw some of them with bare feet). Those who do not mess their pants, or drop from exhaustion are reckoned to be liars, and told to "go back". A protest has been made, and a change is expected in both methods and personnel.'[15]

On 4 June 1943 an unprecedented third Japanese medical 'investigation' was started. On 5 June the prisoners each received what they were informed was an 'Anti-dysentery inoculation. ½cc.' This 'medicine' apparently had the reverse effect on the men, or at least no discernably relieving effect, for three days later Peaty wrote 'Diarrhoea still steadily increasing.'[16] Private Schreiner recorded in his diary that the inoculation was preceded by an examination of both body and mind by a Japanese psychologist and his assistants. Firstly, the height and weight of each prisoner was carefully recorded. Then 'we stripped naked and went into a small room. Here the doctor sat at a desk on the other side of the room and asked a lot of questions. Examples – "Would you like to go home?" "What do you think?" "Are you a peaceful man?"'[17] This lasted for around fifteen minutes before each man received his 'so-called dysentery injection,' wrote Schreiner.

The number of American prisoners who died continued to increase during 1943, and the battery of inoculations that the POWs were subjected to appeared to have no affect against whatever was killing the sick men. This suggests that either all of the Japanese doctors had not managed to isolate and identify what was killing the prisoners, or that the Japanese were incompetent. Considering how many Japanese doctors were involved in three separate investigations into the high mortality rate at Mukden

Camp, the second charge seems unlikely. On the first charge, perhaps it was not so much a question of identifying what was killing the prisoners, but rather a question of what the Japanese *gave* to the prisoners that killed them. Medical investigations conducted in this manner have all the hallmarks of medical *observations* of the course of a disease that had been deliberately introduced to the prisoners. The open-air autopsies already noted to have taken place at Mukden were further evidence of experiments being carried out in the camp, as this follows the standard procedure at Pingfan. No other camp witnessed autopsies being performed on prisoners who had died of disease, even when the numbers of dead were extremely high.

Major Peaty recorded in his diary that as well as regular inoculations, *all* of the prisoners were subjected to regular rectal examinations where doctors inserted glass rods into their anuses. Faecal smears were also taken from the prisoners, and blood tests were occasionally taken. The rectal examinations are revealing from a purely medical point-of-view, and certainly point to some sort of organised observation of the progress of a disease. According to medical experts I spoke to, rectal examinations are still conducted using a similar apparatus, although today it is made of plastic – a procedure called a rigid sigmoidoscopy. It allows the examining physician to see the bottom half of the colon, and any piles, lumps or inflammation that may be present. The faecal smears are taken to look for infections or diseases, as are any blood tests. A rigid sigmoido examination, with associated faecal smear test and blood test, could be used to internally examine a patient who is suffering from dysentery. If these tests were conducted regularly, as Major Peaty and other former Mukden prisoners stated, the doctors may have been tracking how a disease was progressing. It is known from the sources that the Japanese did not prescribe any drugs to alleviate the suffering of the sick prisoners, which would have been the normal procedure after making a physical examination of the patient and a diagnosis. The autopsying of deceased prisoners who apparently died from diarrhoea or dysentery could also be seen as forming a part of any disease study. This was, as mentioned, just the kind of work that was undertaken in the laboratories at Pingfan by Dr. Ishii and his colleagues when they deliberately infected Asian prisoners with a battery of horrible diseases.

Guinea Pigs

Making a link between the unusual medical activities that were recorded inside the Mukden Camp and what was going on at Pingfan has proved difficult, though not as impossible as we have been led to believe by some historians and governments. There is extant documentary evidence that links the Mukden Camp to the activities of Unit 731. A document discovered in the archives of the International Military Tribunal for the Far East (better known as the 'Tokyo Trials'), dated 17 February 1943, records: 'For some purpose unknown, the POWs were sent to this [Mukden] concentration camp. Three months after their arrival, a department chief named Nagayama made a report on the conditions of prisoners and lack of nutrition adjustment in the camp.' The Japanese medical officer named in the report was none other than Dr. Saburo Nagayama, clinical department chief at Unit 731 at Pingfan. If Nagayama had managed to 'make a report' he or his subordinates must have visited the camp, and this indicates that Unit 731 was interested in the prisoners. For such a report to have come from a serving Unit 731 clinician, instead of from a Kwantung Army medic, should be cause for concern. From the statement that Nagayama made, he was concerned that the prisoners at Mukden were not healthy enough, and that action was required to correct this. We can certainly suggest that as the investigation and report originated with a senior Unit 731 doctor, this did not spell good news for the prisoners at Mukden. Perhaps the Japanese had some other agenda apart from restoring the prisoners' health, and that this requirement for healthy prisoners followed the established *modus operandi* at Pingfan exactly.

Japanese documents that survived the war provide more important clues in establishing a link between Mukden Camp and Unit 731. Kwantung Army Operational Order No. 98, issued by the Commander-in-Chief, General Yoshijiro Umezu, is very significant when read alongside other corroborative sources. It reads, in part, 'Assign 32 medical officers to go to the concentration camp for prisoners of war at Mukden.' Could this be the visit by 'About 10 Japanese medical officers, and 20 other ranks ...'[18] noted by Major Robert Peaty in his diary on 13 February 1943? The numbers and timing are very similar. The order to send the thirty-two medical personnel to Mukden was issued on 1 February 1943 by Lieutenant General Ryuji Kajitsuka, Chief of the Medical Department of the Kwantung Army, who had received it down the chain of command from General Umezu. Interestingly, Kajitsuka was Lieutenant General Shiro Ishii's immediate boss.

Before we examine the available witness testimony of former Mukden POWs, there is another extremely interesting source that is worthy of investigation. Some of the most compelling evidence that goes a long way to proving that Unit 731 experimented on POWs at Mukden comes from the Soviet Union. Lieutenant General Kajitsuka was one of twelve Japanese personnel from Unit 731 who had the misfortune to be captured by the Soviets in 1945 and who were later placed on trial in the Siberian city of Khabarovsk between 25 and 30 December 1949. The NKVD, the forerunner of the KGB, had extensively interrogated all twelve of the defendants in the interval between their capture and trial. Their testimony was consistently discounted from investigations into whether Allied POWs were experimented upon by Unit 731, primarily because any Soviet investigation was deemed to have been politically motivated and any statements made by the defendants either forced or drafted for them by the Soviets. The propaganda value of the trial cannot be ignored, but some of the information that emerged from the interrogations was extremely interesting. Discounting the Soviet investigation seems to be historically naïve, given the extensive use of recently opened Soviet archives in Moscow by Western authors investigating the story of the Eastern Front, and particularly the Battle for Berlin and Adolf Hitler's demise in 1945.

The record of the Soviet investigation and trial of the Japanese military personnel stated they fully cooperated with their captors, meaning that they were not tortured in order to extract information. Perhaps, but it does seem reasonable to assume that with the war already lost for Japan, and their biological warfare programme fully stopped, they had little to lose by cooperating. During the war many Allied nations discovered that once Japanese had been taken prisoner, they usually fully cooperated with their captors as their situation placed them beyond the pale of Japanese society who considered death to be the only honourable alternative. The prisoners in Soviet hands would all have been fully aware of the fearsome reputation of the Soviet security police for torture and brutality. Perhaps they hoped to ingratiate themselves with their captors by cooperating. We cannot know for certain. All of the defendants were facing prison for their wartime activities, but

Guinea Pigs

they must also have been aware of their value to the Soviet biological weapons programme. At the same time as they stood trial in Khabarovsk, Shiro Ishii and dozens of their former Unit 731 colleagues, as we will see, were fully collaborating with the Americans in producing even more lethal biological warfare pathogens for use against the Soviet Union.

Two of the defendants placed on trial at Khabarovsk, General Kajitsuka and Major Tomio Karasawa, both admitted to the Soviets that Unit 731 had used Allied POWs in biological warfare experiments in Manchuria. Interestingly, these admissions came freely from the Japanese – the Soviet interrogators were not particularly interested one way or the other. Kajitsuka told the NKVD that Shiro Ishii had spoken to him at length in 1941 on the problems of delivering pathogenic bacteria in aerial bombs to targeted population centres. Specifically, the intention was to spread diseases such as dysentery, typhus, paratyphoid, cholera and bubonic plague by air interdiction, but that in 100 per cent of experiments the bacteria had immediately perished when dropped from aircraft using conventional bombs. Alternatives were sought that eventually produced Ishii's infamous ceramic bombs, a very effective delivery system for disease pathogens. Before this development, Unit 731 experimented with delivering the pathogenic bacteria to human populations in food, specifically in vegetables, fruits, fish and meat. These foods were contaminated with cholera, dysentery, typhus and paratyphoid and then fed to prisoners at Unit 731 and the results carefully studied. Cabbage was discovered to be the most effective carrier of disease bacteria.

Shiro Ishii told Kajitsuka that only by studying human physiological peculiarities would it be possible to obtain knowledge on conditions of artificial arousal of epidemics. Therefore, field-testing was also ordered. 'For instance, there were researches devoted to effects of infecting by pathogenic bacteria humans representing different ethnic groups,' notes Russian historian B.G. Yudin in his examination of the Khabarovsk Trial. 'Along with humans of Chinese, Russian, Korean, Mongolian origin there were experiments on American prisoners of war.'[19] Major Tomio Kawasawa, the other defendant at Khabarovsk who mentioned experiments on Allied POWs in court, was a section chief at Unit 731. Asked by the Soviet state prosecutor, 'Whether Unit 731 was occupied with study of immunity of American prisoners of war to contagious diseases?' Karasawa replied: 'As I can recall, it was in the beginning of 1943.' This date ties in with the worst period of diarrhoea and dysentery at the Mukden Camp, and the highest death toll among the American prisoners. 'At that time I was in a hospital in Mukden and research fellow Minata came to see me,' stated Karasawa in 1949. 'He told me about his work and informed me that at the moment he was in Mukden to study [the] issue of immunity of American prisoners of war.' The prosecutor then asked: 'And for that purpose study of characteristics of blood of American prisoners of war was carried out?' Karasawa replied: 'Just so.'[20] Frustratingly, the Soviet prosecutor did not push Karasawa for more details of the experiments that were undertaken on the Mukden POWs, largely because the Soviets were not that interested.

The issue of 'study of characteristics of blood' of Allied POWs is not particularly sinister, for the Americans also undertook a study of blood serum from German and Japanese POWs. In a different version of the courtroom exchange noted above, the Chinese newspaper *The Beijing Bright Daily* reported Major Karasawa as saying: 'Blood of human species of all peoples was tested for the study of immunity. Minato, a researcher, was sent to study the blood of American POWs.'[21] Could it have been the case that the large number of Japanese doctors and medics who visited Mukden Camp allegedly to investigate the causes of the diarrhoea and dysentery outbreak were actually investigating and recording the results of the deliberate infection of the prisoners? Major Peaty has provided a detailed list of all of the inoculations and tests that he and his men underwent while prisoners at Mukden, and it was a veritable battery of them. Could it not be the case that some of these 'inoculations' were actually making the prisoners sick?

Major Peaty notes the following medical treatments in his diary, and it is transcribed verbatim:

'30 Jan 43   – ½cc mixed Typhoid and Para "A".'
'5 Feb 43   – 1cc mixed Typhoid and Para "A".'
'14 Feb 43   – Vaccination.'
'6 Jun 43   – ½cc Anti-Dysentery innoc. incl. Flechner Y.'
'13 Jun 43   – 1cc Anti-Dysentery innoc. incl. Flechner Y.'
'29 Aug 43   – 1cc T.A.B. (strength unknown).'
'19 Sep 43   – X-ray for TB, Sedimentation Test, Sputum – Test, Mantoux Reaction Test.'

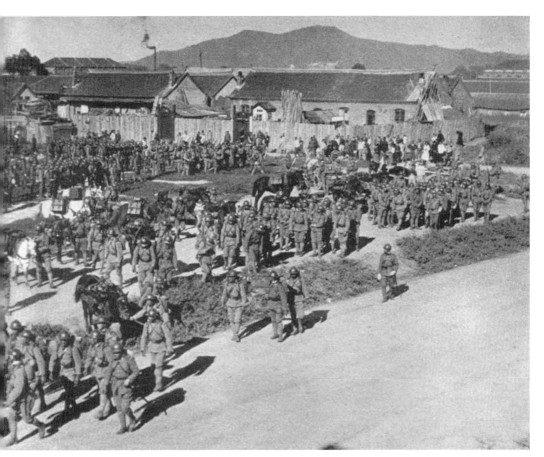

1. Japanese troops massing outside of the city of Mukden (now Shenyang), China, following the infamous 18 September 1931 'Incident'. Shortly after, Manchuria was occupied by Japan and the path to Unit 731 began.

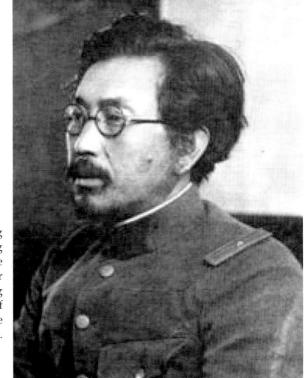

2. Dr Shiro Ishii, pictured here as a young army doctor. The mastermind and driving force behind Japan's biological warfare programme, Ishii escaped prosecution for war crimes in 1945 despite being responsible for hundreds of thousands of deaths and went to work for the Americans.

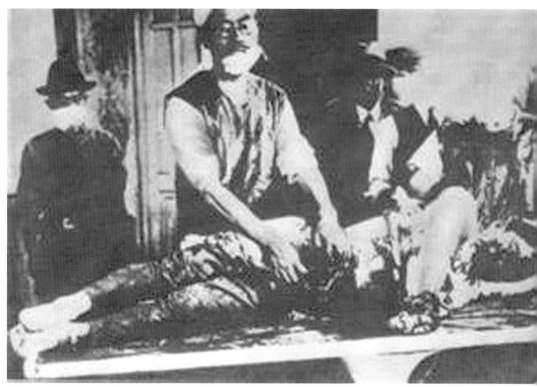

3. A human dissection graphically recorded at Unit 731's main facility outside Pingfan, Manchuria.

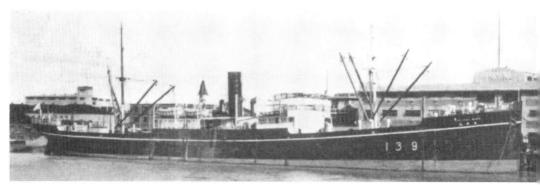

4. The hellship *Tottori Maru*, on which the Japanese transported American prisoners from the Philippines to Manchuria in 1942.

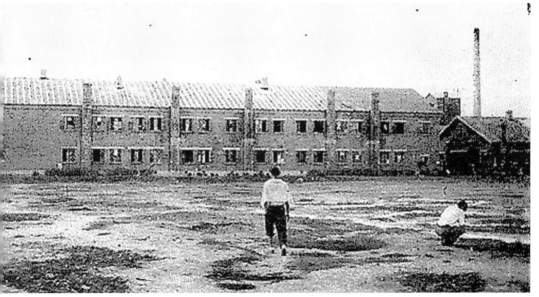

5. One of the prisoner accommodation barracks at Mukden Camp.

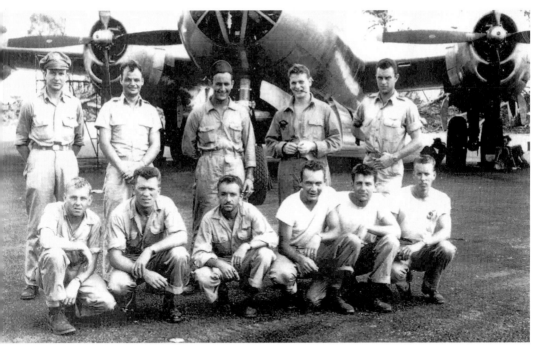

6. Some of the crew of the B-29 shot down over Japan on 5 May 1945. It included eight USAAF airmen who were dissected alive by Japanese doctors at Kyushu Imperial University in Fukuoka. Some of their organs were later cooked and eaten by Japanese officers.

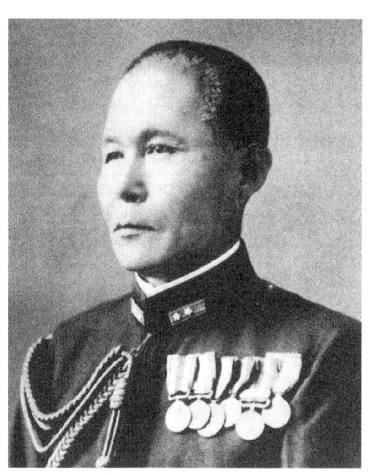

7. Vice Admiral Jisaburo Ozawa. In 1945, as Japan was losing the war, Ozawa hatched a plan called Operation 'PX' with Shiro Ishii to attack the United States with 'germ bombs' developed at Unit 731.

8. Allied prisoners of war shortly after the liberation of Mukden Camp by units of the Red Army, August 1945.

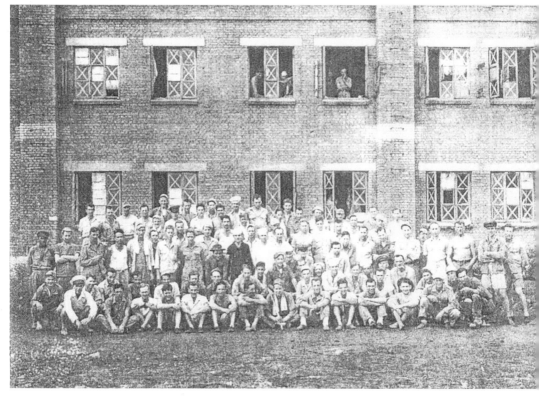

9. American POW John Parsons photographed at Mukden Camp with two of his Soviet liberators, August 1945.

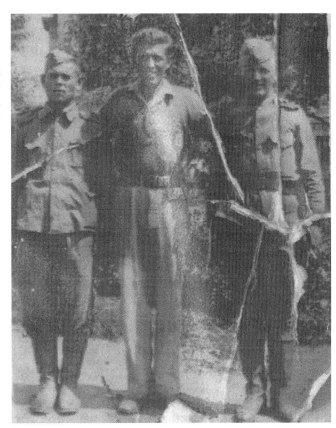

10. USAAF airmen pictured shortly after their release from Mukden Camp, August 1945.

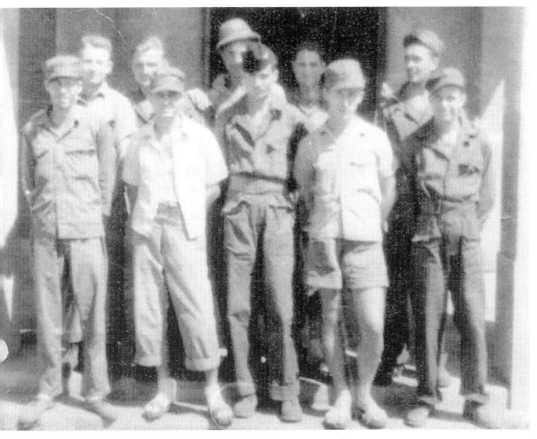

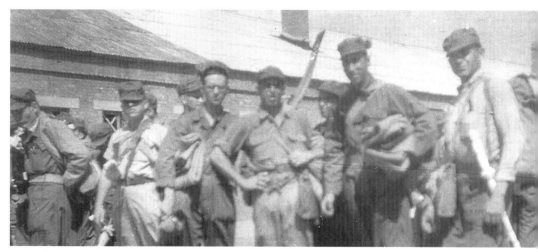

11. Liberated Allied POWs prepare to evacuate Mukden Camp, September 1945.

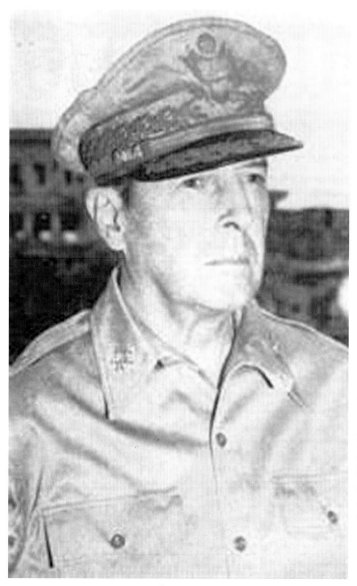

12. General Douglas MacArthur, postwar Governor of Japan. He urged the American government to grant Ishii and his associates immunity from prosecution for war crimes in return for gaining secret data derived from Japan's biological and chemical warfare experiments on humans, including Allied POWs.

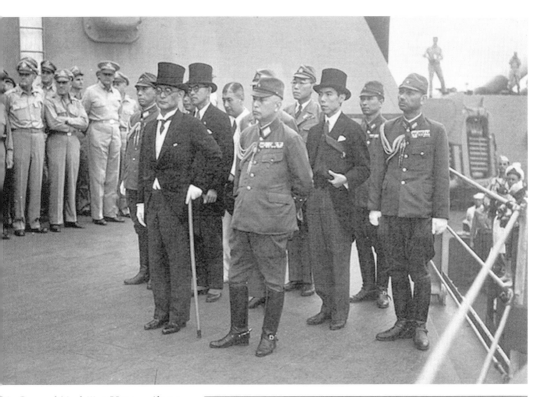

13. General Yoshijiro Umezu (front row, right), photographed at the official surrender of Japan aboard the USS *Missouri* in Tokyo Bay. Umezu prevented Admiral Ozawa's Operation 'PX' from being carried out, and probably saved tens of thousands of American lives.

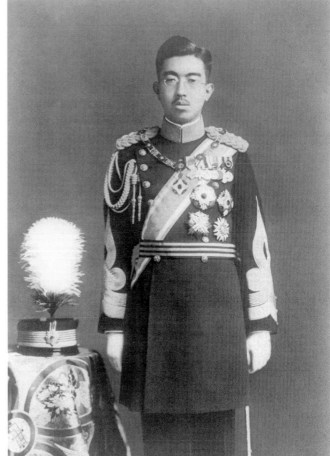

14. Emperor Hirohito of Japan. Close links have been suggested between Hirohito, members of the Imperial Family and Unit 731.

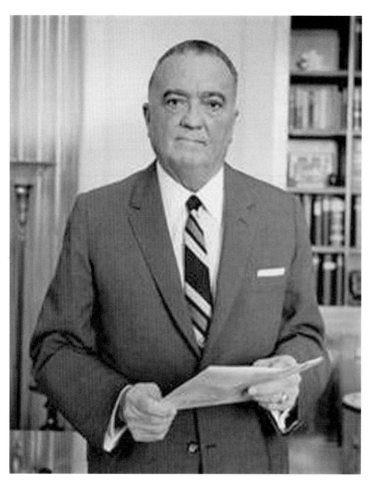

15. FBI Director J. Edgar Hoover. In 1956 he sent agents to investigate claims that American and Allied POWs had been experimented on by Unit 731 personnel during the war. The FBI was denied access to this information.

16. Unit 731 today, a sobering reminder of the level of brutality during the Japanese occupation of China.

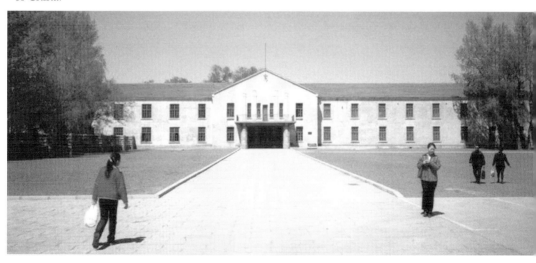

Guinea Pigs

'10 Oct 43   – ½cc Cholera innoc.'
'17 Oct 43   – 1cc Cholera innoc.'
'6 Feb 44   – Vaccination of the whole camp.'
'20 Feb 44   – ½cc T.A.B. innoc.'
'27 Feb 44   – 1cc T.A.B. innoc. (39.36% infected).'
'7 Mar 44   – Stool test for round worms.'
'21 May 44   – ½cc Anti-Dysentery innoc.'
'28 May 44   – 1cc Anti-Dysentery innoc.'
'20 Aug 44   – 1cc T.A.B. inoculation for everyone.'
'28 Jan 45   – Vaccination for everyone.'
'27 Feb 45   – ½cc T.A.B. innoc.'
'6 Mar 45   – 1cc T.A.B.'

Available witness testimony, apart from the diaries already discussed and the reports of the senior American and British officers who were imprisoned at Mukden, has come from a handful of American enlisted men who appeared before the US House of Representatives Veterans' Affairs Subcommittee meetings of 1982 and 1986 respectively. The rest were veterans who were interviewed in the 1990s by the American historian Linda Goetz Holmes. The witnesses all said they had been the victims of Japanese human medical experiments, and those who appeared before Congress sought financial compensation from a resistant American government. All of the men described constant hunger and malnutrition as being a major part of their experiences at Mukden from the time of their arrival at the temporary camp in November 1942 until their liberation from the permanent 'Hoten' camp in August 1945. Of interest to us is whether the officers' diaries and reports written at the time, particularly Major Peaty's blow-by-blow account of imprisonment at Mukden, corroborate anything the veterans said at their hearings which concerned supposed medical experiments being conducted by the Japanese, and whether they also corroborate the Japanese assertions made during the Khabarovsk War Crimes Trial.

According to one American veteran, Frank James, the Japanese medical tests actually began in Pusan, Korea, shortly after the transport ship bringing them from the Philippines docked, as will be discussed shortly. Before the prisoners were processed on arrival at Mukden Camp on 11 November 1942 a team of Japanese physicians conducted further tests. James told Linda Holmes:

'Everybody had six or seven blood samples taken. All of us at Mukden were directly or indirectly used for experiments. I had constant diarrhea. Medical data was being constantly taken by Japanese doctors.'[22] We know that dead Americans were autopsied on site at the Mukden temporary camp by a team of Japanese Army surgeons and medics because Major Peaty recorded this fact in his diary on 15 February 1943 when he wrote: 'Autopsies being performed on the corpses by the visiting Japanese.'[23] In 1986 Frank James testified before Congress that he had actually assisted the Japanese doctors during the autopsies of American prisoners who had died during the winter of 1942–43 and because the ground was frozen solid, their corpses were stored in a wooden shed at the camp until the spring. James had been assigned to the burial details shortly after his arrival at the camp. By the spring of 1943 James and his colleagues had over two hundred bodies to bury. 'A team of Japanese medical personnel, Unit 731, arrived with an autopsy table for taking specimens,' James said. Along with another American prisoner, James was given the task of lifting the bodies off the table. 'Those bodies had been selected ... Then the Japanese opened the bodies – the head, chest and stomach – and took out the desired specimens, which were placed in containers and marked with the POWs' numbers.'[24]

Another veteran, Warren W. Whelchel from Oklahoma, stated in 1982: 'Some persons were checked for oral and rectal temperatures, some for whelps the shots caused, rectal tissues for some, rectal smears from others. All the personnel were sprayed in the face by some kind of spray from a spray instrument similar to our Flit spray guns.'[25] According to Whelchel this was only done to a segregated group of American prisoners that was then permitted to integrate with the other prisoners. 'The Japanese medical personnel were keeping accurate records of each and every one of us in this one barracks,'[26] stated Whelchel. Five or six Japanese doctors had interviewed the selected American prisoners. Sheldon H. Harris, author of *Factories of Death* states: 'The doctors gave the Americans various shots discriminately; not all the prisoners were given the same type of shots.'[27] Warren Whelchel also testified: 'We felt that we were being tested for bacteriological immunity for their possible use of bacterial warfare against the Allied troops in the Far East.' Perhaps, but Whelchel's statement seems to have been influenced by post-war hindsight. Certainly neither Major

Guinea Pigs

Peaty, nor imprisoned American doctor Captain Mark Herbst, came to this strong conclusion whilst actually in the camp in 1943. In 1982 veteran Gregory Rodriguez testified that he had suffered from episodic and chronic illness for decades since his imprisonment at Mukden – and he associated the illness with the placing of a feather under his nose by Japanese medics. He also recalled opening Red Cross packages and discovering numerous feathers of various colours that had been placed amongst the food items. The Japanese did use infected feathers as a way of spreading pathogens at Unit 731 in Pingfan, and perhaps the different colours used indicated some secret cataloguing or coding system for the test. Other prisoners recalled the same use of feathers by the Japanese, including veteran W. Wesley Davis, who told Linda Holmes: 'I was asleep on a straw mat on the platform (our bed) in our barracks. At about 4 a.m. I was awakened by a tickling sensation. I awoke with a start to see the face of a Japanese unfamiliar to me holding a feather under my nose. When I awoke, he quickly said "excuse me" and moved away before I could ask what he was doing.'[28] Other former POWs who were interviewed by Holmes also recalled feathers, and in some instances, the Japanese placing tags marked with numbers onto their toes, as they lay asleep.

Rodriguez's son Gregory Jr. testified before Congress in 1986 after his father had passed away stating that his father's illness included fever, pain and fatigue, and that an American doctor confirmed the veteran was suffering from recurrent typhoid. A blood test revealed a large number of typhoid bacteria still in his blood. Of course, it is impossible to demonstrate any evidentiary chain existing between the claims of Rodriguez father and son and the Mukden Camp.

Veteran Frank James of California corroborated many of the claims made by Warren Whelchel when he testified before the Congressional Sub-Committee in 1986. James stated that when the prisoners arrived at the camp on 11 November 1942 a team of Japanese medics, who were wearing facemasks, met them. These Japanese proceeded to spray a 'liquid in our faces and we were given injections.' When they had been en route to Mukden from Pusan in Korea 'we had glass rods inserted in our rectums,'[29] recalled James, the rigid sigmoidoscopies referred to earlier that permitted an examination of the lower colon. The team of mysterious Japanese medical personnel was reported by several independent witnesses, including Major Peaty, who noted in his diary on 13 February 1943: 'About 10 Japanese medical officers, and 20 other ranks ... arrived to-day to investigate the cause of the large number of deaths.'[30] US Army Air Corps veteran Robert Brown, who worked as a medical technician in the Mukden Camp hospital, recalled the arrival of a team of Japanese personnel who wore white smocks and masks. They injected some of the prisoners, and prevented the burial detail from doing their jobs until autopsies had been performed on some of the bodies, a fact that was corroborated by Frank James, who had actually been a member of the burial detail at Mukden. 'I don't know what medical facility they came from,' stated Brown. 'All I know is they arrived by truck, they were in medical garb, and they were not part of the Japanese medical staff at our POW camp, and they visited the facility several times.'[31] Another American prisoner, Art Campbell, stated: 'A crew of Japanese we hadn't seen before lined us up. They were dressed in white and gave each of us half an orange. Two or three days later, everybody was very sick. I had a high fever. Later, we figured out the oranges must have been doctored with something. I know I'd have eaten it anyway because I had scurvy so bad.'[32] As already noted, Peaty had carefully recorded the distribution of oranges to the prisoners in his diary. Campbell recalled how the Japanese treated the men who had received the oranges: 'They took nine of us and put us in a special ward. They tested our blood, everything. They started giving us shots regularly, 500cc's at a time, and said it was horse urine and would be good for us because it had vitamin C in it.'[33] As will be seen in the next chapter the use of horse urine in human experiments was not limited to Mukden.

Many historians have chosen to either doubt or discard the eye-witness testimonies that were recorded before Congress in the 1980s, seeing them as unreliable, exaggerated, vague, or, in the case of Rodriguez Jr., third-person. Any police officer or barrister knows that witness testimony often is all of those things, but when enough witnesses are saying the same things, a pattern of truth emerges. The testimonies of James, Whelchel and Rodriguez Senior either indicate that these men had fantastic imaginations, or that they had, indeed, witnessed unusual medical practices going on at the Mukden Camp that they, with their lack of medical knowledge, could not fully comprehend. When the testimonies of the men that Linda Goetz Holmes spoke to are included in the story, it becomes compelling. Holmes made the point that none of the men she spoke to were specifically interviewed concerning possible Japanese medical experiments – rather these men all *volunteered* this information unprompted during the course of the interviews. Parts of these oral testimonies have been verified from the extant documentation – for example, Frank James' assertion of autopsies at Mukden Camp is borne out by Major Peaty's contemporary record, and therefore it is undeniably true. Holmes says in her book that she takes the journalist's rule of thumb: 'If several sources, independent of one another, tell the same story, it has a certain amount of credibility. Especially if the individuals are not interviewed at the same time, or at the same gathering.' Holmes is in no doubt that the medical history of Mukden Camp was unusual, to say the least: 'After interviewing dozens of ex-POWs from the Mukden complex, it seems apparent to this writer that on several occasions, medical personnel from elsewhere were allowed to visit the POW hospital and some barracks at the Mitsubishi Mukden camps, and that after they left, a certain number of POWs became very ill or subsequently died in a short time.'[34]

In 1986 Frank James corroborated Major Tomio Kawasawa's 1949 courtroom admission that Unit 731 doctors were interested in testing the 'immunity of Anglo-Saxons' to diseases. James claimed visiting teams of Japanese medical personnel questioned the Americans about their ethnic backgrounds and demanded specific information. 'It had to be Scotch, French, English, or whatever,'[35] said James. The American veteran claimed the doctors who questioned him and his comrades about their racial ancestry were the same doctors he had been forced to assist at the aforementioned autopsies. The doctors performed 'what seemed to be a psycho-physical and anatomical examination on selected POWs. I was one of them.'[36] James recalled the prisoners were 'required to walk in footsteps that had been painted on the floor, which led to a desk, at which the Japanese medical personnel sat.' James and his comrades were then closely questioned regarding their backgrounds. The Japanese doctors also 'measured my head, shoulders, arms and legs with calipers, and asked many questions about the medical history of my family.'[37] James claims he and other American prisoners who experienced these tests did not come forward about what had happened to them for several decades after the war because the US Army had forced them to sign a pledge not to talk about their experiences 'under threat of court martial.'[38]

Turning now to the surviving evidence from the Japanese themselves, much of this evidence rather neatly corroborates what American and British sources have already stated. Japanese Unit 731 veteran Tsuneji Shimada recalled in 1985 that a Dr. 'Minato', a name very close to the Japanese research fellow at Mukden Military Hospital surnamed 'Minata' who was identified by Major Tomio Karasawa during the course of the 1949 Khabarovsk War Crimes Trial was intimately involved with the Mukden Camp. Karasawa said in 1949: 'At that time [early 1943] I was in a hospital in Mukden and research fellow Minata came to see me. He told me about his work and informed me that at the moment he was in Mukden to study [the] issue of immunity of American prisoners of war.'[39] Tsuneji Shimada stated in 1985 that Dr. Minato performed tests on American POWs at Mukden Camp using dysentery bacteria. Shimada claimed that Minato ordered blood tests to be taken from the prisoners, that selected prisoners were given liquids to drink which had been infected with dysentery bacteria, and that some of those who died were subjected to autopsies in order to assess the internal effects of the bacteria. Major Peaty noted the presence of a large group of Japanese medical personnel in the camp on 13 February 1943. Peaty's figure of thirty Japanese medics and the date closely equates to Kwantung Army Operational Order No. 98, issued by Commander-in-chief General Yoshijiro Umezu. It read, in part, 'Assign 32 medical officers to go to the concentration camp for prisoners of war at Mukden.' Lieutenant General Ryuji Kajitsuka, the aforementioned chief of the medical department of the Kwantung Army, signed off on this order on 1 February 1943.

More evidence emerged after the war from the American side. In 1956, an FBI agent investigating whether Allied – and specifically American – POWs had been the victims of biological warfare experiments by the Japanese sent a memorandum to Director J. Edgar Hoover in Washington D.C. The memo, dated 13 March, detailed the agent's meeting with James J. Kellehar, Jr., from the Office of Special Operations, Department of Defense. The agent

Guinea Pigs

stated that Kelleher 'has volunteered further comments to the effect that American Military Forces after occupying Japan, determined that the Japanese actually did experiment with "BW" [biological warfare] agents in Manchuria during 1943–44 *using American prisoners as test victims* [author's emphasis]'[40]. Intriguingly, the FBI agent went on to state that '... information of the type in question is closely controlled and regarded as highly sensitive.' Closely controlled by whom? Sensitive to whom? As will be revealed later, the wartime research and activities of Shiro Ishii and his colleagues at Unit 731 became of primary importance to the United States military after the war, and was the subject of a grubby backstairs deal between Cold War intelligence assets and the Japanese that granted these war criminals immunity from prosecution in return for their biological warfare secrets. The 1956 memo demonstrated that even an agency as powerful as Hoover's FBI could not penetrate the ring of silence that surrounded how the Americans had obtained their immense lead in biological warfare technology – and it also goes some way to explaining why researchers today are unable to definitively answer the question of whether Allied POWs were subjected to experiments at the Mukden Camp, as the relevant documents are probably, in the words of the FBI agent, 'controlled and regarded as highly sensitive.'

The author Sheldon H. Harris, who quotes the 1956 FBI memo in *Factories of Death*, attaches no significance to it whatsoever, which is rather astounding. In my opinion the memo is one of the most significant extant documents to address the question of Allied POW experimentation, and it also provides an interesting link with a secret US Army operation codenamed 'Flamingo' that was thrown together during the dying days of the war to retrieve secret documentation from Pingfan. This covert and highly significant operation has also similarly been overlooked or sidelined by historians, and will be dealt with later.

Before moving on to examine the American cover-up of Unit 731's activities in Manchuria, it is necessary to try and discover which diseases the Japanese doctors were likely experimenting with at the Mukden POW Camp. It has been well documented that researchers at Unit 731 were interested in several specific diseases; a list that prominently included bubonic plague, typhoid, paratyphoid, glanders, cholera and dysentery. We can probably discount some of the diseases listed above immediately from the experiments undertaken at Mukden Camp as their obvious and pronounced symptoms would have been noted by prisoner doctor Captain Mark Herbst in his report cited extensively in the previous chapter, concerning the medical conditions inside the camp, or else have appeared in the diary of the Australian doctor Captain Brennan.

The bubonic plague, known in Europe as the 'Black Death', was quite common in Asia well into the twentiethth century and it was certainly one of the central areas of Dr. Shiro Ishii's biological weapons research at Pingfan. The Japanese wanted to use it against the Chinese population. The symptoms of the plague include painful and swollen lymph glands in the armpits, groin or neck, accompanied by chills, malaise, a high fever of 39 degrees Celsius, muscle pain, severe headache and heavy breathing. Other symptoms include the continuous vomiting of blood, the urination of blood, coughing, extreme pain all over the body, and lenticulae (black dots scattered throughout the body – hence the name 'Black Death') – delirium and coma. None of the prisoners appear to have exhibited these symptoms. Another disease, which based on the witness testimony can be ruled out, is typhoid fever, another major research area for Unit 731 physicians at Pingfan. Typhoid manifests itself as a slow progressive fever that may rise as high as 40 degrees Celsius, accompanied by profuse sweating and gastroenteritis. The disease progresses in four distinctly awful stages over a period of four weeks, and can be fatal if left untreated. In week one the patient's temperature slowly rises, and a cough, headache, and a feeling of general malaise, accompany this. By week two the patient is prostrated, suffering from a high fever, bradycardia (slow heart rate), and delirium. The abdomen is distended with pain in the extreme right lower quadrant. The sufferer passes between six and eight stools a day in the form of pea-green stinking diarrhoea, or conversely, in some cases the patient may be constipated. The spleen and liver may also be enlarged. In week three intestinal haemorrhage or perforation may occur, as well as neuropsychiatric symptoms. In week four the person either recovers or dies. Based on Captain Herbst's medical observations, such severe symptoms as would normally be associated with typhoid fever do not appear to be present in the ill prisoners, and this is confirmed by an examination of Major Peaty's diary and Major Hankins' report.

There is a disease with somewhat similar symptoms to typhoid which could be a possible candidate, based on symptoms among the prisoners that were noted by contemporary witnesses. Paratyphoid fever is more benign that typhoid. It is an enteric, or digestive tract, illness caused by strains of the bacterium *Salmonella paratyphi* and is divided into three different species, A, B or C. Paratyphoid is transmitted by means of contaminated food or water, hence the interest of Unit 731 scientists in it. It is interesting to note that some of the American witnesses spoke of being given food they felt had been doctored by the Japanese – particularly small oranges – or of finding coloured feathers inside their Red Cross food parcels. Others recalled being sprayed in the face by some unknown substance and receiving injections of yet more unidentified solutions. However, paratyphoid can probably also be discounted in the case of the Mukden Camp because its symptoms do not match most of what has been reported. Paratyphoid causes a sustained fever, a headache, abdominal pain, malaise, anorexia, cough, and bradycardia. The spleen or the liver may also be enlarged as with typhoid fever. In Caucasians, studies have shown that 30 per cent will develop rosy spots on the central body (a fact never reported or noted by any of the witnesses at the Mukden Camp), and constipation is much more common than diarrhoea. Dysentery and diarrhoea were the main symptoms reported by the witnesses at Mukden Camp – apparently in epidemic proportions judging from the casualty rate and the state of the latrines.

The level of diarrhoea reported by the witnesses at the Mukden Camp suggests that if the Japanese were testing a bacterium on POWs, it was most probably a strain of dysentery, an extremely common disease in developing countries, and a common complaint among Allied soldiers who fought against the Japanese. My grandfather recalled the exhaustion of suffering from both dysentery and malaria at the same time whilst fighting the Japanese in the Burmese jungle in 1945, and any examination of conditions inside Japanese POW camps showed high levels of dysentery usually caused by a lack of proper sanitation. Japanese troops in the field were as equally prone to dysentery as British and American troops, and the myth that the Japanese soldier was somehow better adapted to conditions in the jungle than his Caucasian or Indian adversary was just that – a myth. In many cases, Japanese troops were in a worse condition than Allied soldiers owing to their army's much more primitive medical supply situation and an inability to properly feed their troops in the field.

Dysentery is an inflammatory disorder of the intestines, particularly of the colon, which causes severe diarrhoea. Mucus and/or blood are usually found in the faeces, and the patient often suffers concurrently with a fever and abdominal pain. Not everyone will develop dysentery when exposed to the bacteria, and some may experience mild or no symptoms whatsoever, whereas others will be severely ill. If left untreated, dysentery can kill, particularly if the patient is unable to rehydrate properly after passing so much liquid. This was a problem for British troops on campaign who maintained a severe form of water discipline when in the field that has since been proved to be unsafe and abandoned by the British Army. A lack of clean drinking water can further compound the problem and leave the sufferer open to other infections, such as typhoid or cholera.

Dysentery is commonly spread through unclean food or water. Two main types exist, bacillary and amoebic, and doctors test for the disease by making cultures of stool samples. Blood tests can be used to measure abnormalities in the levels of essential minerals and salts in the body. An examination of the patient's colon by rigid sigmoidoscopy would tell the examining doctor how far the disease had progressed, coupled with a blood test and faecal smear test. It could have been that the Japanese were testing to see how the dysentery would spread among the prisoners by infecting one small group – the 'segregated' group that was spoken of by veterans Warren Whelchel and Frank James in their US Congressional testimony – and then permit them to freely mix with the rest of the prisoner population. Regular tests were then conducted on all of the prisoners in an attempt to see if the 'Anglo-Saxons' had a resistance to certain strains of the disease by working out the percentage that became sick at different times during the course of the study. The autopsies witnessed by Major Peaty and Frank James made scientific sense to the Japanese because they would have wanted to determine the extent of the infection inside Caucasian prisoners who had actually died, and compare that data with what they already knew about Asians from their secret tests at Pingfan and elsewhere. I surmise that for any such study to successfully isolate which strain of dysentery was most lethal against Caucasians, the Japanese would have tested all of the various strains at different times – hence the fact that although the Japanese claimed they were treating the successive diarrhoea outbreaks at the Mukden Camp by dispatching large teams of medical personnel to 'investigate', they were in reality only infecting and testing the prisoners for their immunity. This is probably why several witnesses, including Captain Herbst and Major Peaty, noted that the Japanese refused to distribute medicines to cure the rampant diarrhoea. The introduction of drugs would have interfered with the test results, and rendered the experiment a waste of time and effort.

Chapter 7

Precedents and Paper Trails

Into the blood steams of POWs Tokada injected mixtures of castor oil and sulphur, of acid, ether and blood plasma. Despite all this, Shinagawa was regarded as a 'showpiece' and was proudly exhibited to visiting Jap generals.

Captain Harold Keschner,
US Army Medical Corps, 1945

'The japs took the excrement [from the latrines], which was full of amoebic dysentery germs, and sprayed it throughout the camp.'[1] Sound familiar? These words were spoken by a former POW, US Army doctor Captain Robert Gottlieb, at the war crimes trial of a Japanese military doctor who stood accused of using Allied soldiers as human guinea pigs in a series of bizarre and lethal medical experiments. The similarity of some of these well-documented experiments to those allegedly undertaken at the Mukden Camp, add a further level of compelling *prima facie* evidence suggesting the involvement of Unit 731 scientists in research on Caucasians.

The question of establishing whether Allied prisoners-of-war were subjected to medical experiments at the Mukden Camp in Manchuria probably can never be conclusively proved or disproved. The documentary evidence necessary for such a firm conclusion simply no longer exists in the public domain, and if it has not already been destroyed, it remains classified to this day in secret military archives in the United States and Japan. Most probably documents that could have settled the question did exist among the several tons of Japanese military papers that were inexplicably returned to Japan in the 1950s by the United States. These documents were not even copied, let alone translated, by American intelligence. Locating where those documents are today in Japan, and gaining access to them is a well nigh impossible task. During the course of the 1986 Congressional hearings concerning allegations of biological warfare experiments at Mukden, the committee called Dr. John Hatcher, Chief of Army Records Management, to try and throw some light onto the topic under discussion. Hatcher claimed he and his colleagues had made an exhaustive search of the files, but had failed to find anything relating to tests conducted on POWs by the Japanese. However, when pressed, Hatcher intriguingly stated: 'It is possible that in one brief period we may have had some of those materials.'[2] Hatcher explained that in 1945 US Army Intelligence had seized a huge amount of Japanese archival material and shipped it to Washington D.C. where it was stored in the National Archives. After a number of years these documents were 'finally boxed up and sent back to Japan,' stated Hatcher, 'because the problem of language was too difficult for us to overcome.'[3] This has to stand as one of the most ridiculous explanations that surround the whole story of Mukden. In a country that contained several million people of Japanese descent, sufficient translators could not be found? 'In fact,' continued Hatcher, 'they [the documents] were so difficult that we did not even copy them.'[4] Naturally, the committee members spend a few astonished moments picking their jaws up off their desks after this admission. This was not just incompetence, but clearly something more sinister. Why were the documents not placed in permanent storage? Why were they not copied? And why were they sent back to the Japanese? Hatcher claimed the decision to send the material back to Japan had been a joint one between the Department of Defense and the State Department. According to historian Sheldon Harris, the pointed questions asked of Hatcher by the sub-committee in 1986 after he had dropped this bombshell into the proceedings, suggested that the committee members believed that 'either the Army was engaged in a cover-up of the charges, or that Army and State Department personnel were unusually inept, or perhaps both.'[5]

So far, the evidence, including American, British and Japanese witness testimonies, Japanese military orders, and an examination of the conditions at the Mukden Camp, all indicate that something was not quite right about this particular POW centre. The treatment of the prisoners held there does not fit in with what we know about most other Japanese camps. The question is; does evidence exist for Japanese medical experiments having been conducted on Allied POWs at any other place except for Mukden? The answer is an emphatic 'yes'. Allied POWs were subjected to fully-documented medical experiments elsewhere in Occupied Asia by Japanese Army units affiliated to Unit 731, and this provides a precedent for assuming, from the available evidence, that the Japanese were doing the same thing at the Mukden Camp.

The most infamous of these documented cases of human experiments on Allied POWs occurred at the Shinagawa Prisoner-of-War Hospital in Tokyo. The use of the word 'hospital' in the title of this facility is rather disingenuous. Built as a labour camp early in the war just outside of Tokyo, it housed British and Australian prisoners from Singapore and Americans from the Philippines. It was a standard run-of-the-mill Japanese POW camp where the inmates were illegally used as forced labourers in various local Japanese businesses until they were moved to a new camp constructed at the town of Omori. The Omori Camp was located on an artificial island in Tokyo Bay, halfway between Tokyo and the port city of Yokohama. The prisoners from Shinagawa were moved there, and Shinagawa redesignated as a 'hospital'. The Japanese used it as a dumping ground for sick prisoners from the many other POW camps that were located throughout the region. It was effectively a facility to hold those who were inevitably going to perish. 'Many a man who was sent to the dirt-floored buildings at Shinagawa, a lone hospital for 8,000 prisoners near Tokyo, simply went to his death,' reported *TIME* magazine in September 1945. 'There was no sanitation; patients slept without blankets on flea-ridden mats. The operating tables were bare board. When the hospital's crematorium was bombed to rubble, prisoners were forced to cremate the dead on spits over an open fire.'[6]

At this camp of the dead, the Japanese decided to use the human material in their hands for a series of immoral medical experiments. The Japanese physician responsible for the cruel medical procedures and experiments that occurred at Shinagawa was later the subject of a war crimes trial convened by the American military, hence the fact that the experiments cannot be denied as everything was openly admitted to in court through detailed cross-examination and witness testimony. Captain Hisikichi Tokada's experiments, if such a word can be applied to what he did, were conducted in full view of many Allied doctors who were labouring under intensely difficult conditions trying to save as many men as they could. These doctors took careful note of what they witnessed, and later testified at Tokada's trial.

Captain Tokada researched a series of diseases, apparently without any proper methodology, causing war crimes prosecutors to label him a 'sadist' who simply enjoyed inflicting pain and suffering upon those under his control. For example, Tokada had POWs who were already suffering from beriberi deliberately infected with different strains of malaria. Tuberculosis patients were injected with concoctions of acid mixed with dextrose, ether or blood plasma, and significant dysentery experiments were undertaken. It is clear that the Japanese military were very interested in the resistance of Caucasians to different strains of dysentery, and this appears to have formed the majority of documented human experimentation conducted using Allied POWs. It is small wonder that the prisoners who were unfortunate enough to have been sent to Shinagawa named Tokada 'The Mad Doctor'.

Captain Robert Gottlieb, who had been captured in the Philippines, recalled the conditions inside the Shinagawa hospital complex, which was to all intents and purposes a grim and badly constructed POW camp. 'Latrines were mere holes in the ground lined with concrete ...'[7] Gottlieb and another US Army doctor, Harold Keschner, stated at Tokada's war crimes trial that they witnessed him inject the infected bile of POWs who were suffering from amoebic dysentery into POWs who were already sick with TB. The historian Daniel Barenblatt suggests in his book *A Plague Upon Humanity* that POWs were also sprayed in the face with dysentery amoebas taken from the camp latrines so that the Japanese could 'farm' those who contracted the organism for experimental drugs derived from their still-living organs. The method of infection is remarkably similar to that alleged to have occurred at the Mukden Camp by several American veterans. According to *TIME* magazine, whose reporter was in Tokyo on 10 September 1945 with the US Navy during the evacuation of Allied POWs from camps around the city, witnesses told the magazine that Captain Tokada and his associates had experimented on them. Captain Keschner, the young army doctor who had been captured at Bataan, said that twenty-nine-year-old Tokada had conducted seemingly insane injection tests, and not only of dysentery. The objective of these tests remains unclear and contemporary witnesses and investigators called the sanity of Dr. Tokada into question. 'Into tubercular men he [Tokada] injected an acid mixed with infected bile. Once he squeezed a milk of ground soy beans into the jugular veins of two men. All died.'[8]

When he was on trial for his life in Tokyo in 1948, Tokada's habit of injecting selected prisoners with soybean protein came up. A witness recalled the sad fate of a British merchant mariner named William Holland whom Tokada experimented on. 'Holland's legs jumped and his mouth foamed in howling idiocy before he died.'[9] Captain Keschner reported: 'Into the blood streams of others he [Tokada] injected mixtures of castor oil and sulphur, of acid, ether and blood plasma. Despite all this, Shinagawa was regarded as a 'showpiece' and was proudly exhibited to visiting Jap generals.'[10] Unlike his medical colleagues in Unit 731 in Manchuria, Captain Tokada at Shinagawa Hospital was found guilty of the charges arrayed against him in Tokyo in 1948 and sentenced to death. He was hanged soon after; an act that many felt provided some small measure of justice for his numerous victims.

Elsewhere in Asia, released Allied POWs began to speak of human medical experimentation from several different locales. Some of these were well-documented cases and the Japanese personnel responsible were brought to trial and punished. At the township of Rabaul in Papua New Guinea, Australian, New Zealand and American POWs were used in malaria and malnutrition experiments conducted by the Rabaul Water Purification Unit, a Japanese Army medical unit directly linked with Unit 731 in Manchuria. The unit was under the command of Captain Einosuke Hirano. Some of the prisoners held at Rabaul died after being injected with malaria-infected human blood.

On Hainan, a large island just off the southern Chinese coast, Australian and Dutch POWs were used in a horrific vitamin experiment. The prisoners were fed a diet that was carefully devoid of certain essential vitamins, including being served with polished rice. Japanese military doctors noted the resulting severe

Precedents and Paper Trails

malnutrition. Many of the prisoners only survived by secretly catching and eating the rats that abounded throughout their camp.

As for the prisoners at Mukden, the strange deaths from an apparent strain of dysentery continued throughout most of the rest of the war. On 12 November 1944 the POWs at Mukden were suddenly joined by 246 new arrivals. These were the senior American, British and Australian officers, their aides, batmen and cooks who had been captured during 1941–42. This group included Lieutenant-General Jonathan Wainwright, the former US commander in the Philippines, and Lieutenant-General Arthur Percival, British commander-in-chief in Malaya. They had been transferred from camps in Formosa where they had been ill treated and humiliated at every turn by the Japanese. The Japanese moved this group to a new branch camp established 100 miles north of Mukden called Hoten Branch Camp No. 1, keeping them away from the original Mukden Camp and its sick inmates. On 1 December 1944 the thirty-four most senior Allied officer prisoners, as well as their aides and batmen, were transferred to Hoten Branch Camp No. 2 that was located close to Liaoyuan in present day Jilin Province.

On 7 December 1944 the Americans mounted a bombing raid on Mukden's industrial centre. The Japanese had illegally sited the Mukden Camp (as well as many of the branch camps) in the midst of heavy industry. Close to the camp was an ammunition factory, tank factory, aircraft factory and a major rail yard, all of which were legitimate Allied targets. The ammunition factory next to the camp was destroyed in the raid, and two bombs fell within the camp perimeter. Nineteen POWs were killed, including the first two British soldiers to die at Mukden; Lance-Bombardier Scholl of the Royal Artillery, who was killed instantly, and Lance-Sergeant Gooby, 2nd Battalion, The Loyal Regiment, who lost a leg and died of his wounds three days later on 10 December. A further thirty POWs were wounded, many of them seriously. On 9 December, after pressure from Majors Hankins and Peaty and the medical officers, the Japanese finally relented and released medicines from the embargoed Red Cross parcels, which undoubtedly saved many lives.

On 21 December 1944 the American B-29s returned and bombed central Mukden again. Some aircraft were downed, and fourteen American airmen were held at Mukden Camp as prisoners until the Japanese surrender. On 29 April 1945 another fresh batch of prisoners was brought into the camp. These were 134 survivors of the sinking of the Japanese hellship *Oryoku Maru* that had fallen victim to an Allied submarine. The prisoners were in a very poor condition on arrival after extensive abuse and maltreatment from the Japanese.

At the Hoten Branch Camp No.1, which was full of brigadiers, colonels and aides, trouble was brewing in May 1945. When ordered to perform manual labour in the fields, the senior Allied officers flatly refused, stating correctly that it was against the terms of the Geneva Convention for officers to perform manual work. In response, the Japanese closed the camp on 20 May and moved the 320 prisoners back to the Mukden Camp.

Even though the war was rapidly coming to a bloody conclusion, the Japanese continued to experiment on Allied POWs. A series of experiments conducted on American prisoners-of-war held in Japan became infamous. There is no dispute over what occurred and it is concrete evidence of widespread interest in Caucasian prisoners by Japanese researchers. The experiments carried out at Kyushu Imperial University in Fukuoka plumbed the very depths of medical depravity and, unusually, resulted in doctors being brought to trial and punished for their actions.

The story began with the shooting down of an American bomber on 5 May 1945. The B-29 Superfortress of the 6th Bomb Squadron, 29th Bomb Group, was part of a fifty-five ship raid on Tachirai Airfield on Kyushu Island from Guam. Three American aircraft were downed by the weak Japanese defences, including one piloted by 1st Lieutenant Marvin Watkins. A Japanese fighter actually rammed Watkins' huge plane, causing sufficient damage for him to give the order to the crew to bail out near the town of Taketa. Hitting the silk over Japan was about the last thing anyone wanted to do as it was tantamount to a death sentence. Since the famous Doolittle Raid on Tokyo in 1942, the Japanese had decreed that all enemy fliers were 'war criminals' and could be dealt with accordingly. What this usually meant was a visit to a kangaroo court, followed by a death sentence, or a lengthy term of harsh imprisonment, all of this interspersed with some torture or other humiliation. In one famous case, airmen from a downed American aircraft were displayed naked in cages at a city zoo for the amusement of locals.

Precedents and Paper Trails

All of the above assumed that the airman actually survived his first few minutes on Japanese soil. Japanese civilians routinely murdered downed aircrew, stabbing or beating them to death, or stringing them up from the nearest tree or lamp-post. Those that were rescued quickly by the *Kempeitai*, the much-feared Japanese military police, faced torture as the Japanese tried to extract military secrets and aircraft data from them. Aboard Watkins' B-29, all eleven crewmen successfully exited the stricken machine and began to descend to earth under their white parachutes. The crewmen were widely dispersed when they hit the ground, and their fates were wildly different.

One American died before reaching the earth after another circling Japanese fighter used its wing to sever his parachute lines. Another landed safely, only to see a mob of baying villagers running towards him armed with a variety of sharp farm implements and sticks. He quickly dragged out his Colt .45 pistol and began firing at them, carefully counting off each round. When he had fired all but one bullet he calmly put the gun to his right temple and pulled the trigger. For a young and healthy man to have chosen so radical a solution as instant suicide gives one an idea of the fear of capture by the Japanese. Another American landed and was shot to death by another enraged crowd of Japanese civilians. The fate of one airman remains unsolved, while the B-29's skipper, 1st Lieutenant Watkins, landed safely and managed to avoid capture for eight hours. The rest of his crew was quickly captured by Japanese Army and *Kempeitai* troops, but not before being badly knocked about by the locals. Some had been stabbed. All were denied any medical treatment and taken instead to a temporary POW centre at Western Army HQ in Fukuoka. A handful of other American airmen shot down earlier were also imprisoned at the centre.

On 17 May a truck took eight of the American aircrew to the Medical Department of the prestigious Kyushu Imperial University in the city, the very institution that counted amongst it alumnus none other than Dr. Shiro Ishii. 1st Lieutenant Watkins was not among them. As the commander of the aircraft and the senior officer who had been captured, the *Kempeitai* shipped him off to Tokyo for a detailed interrogation that involved some torture. He survived the war. Those of his men left behind were turned over to the custody of the doctors and scientists at the university to use as they saw fit. It appears from the trial proceedings that a local Japanese colonel and a medical officer decided to release eight Americans to Kyushu University for the express purpose of human experimentation. The Americans had absolutely no idea of what the Japanese were about to do to them.

The eight American POWs were used in a series of experiments – all of them fatal – overseen by senior Japanese civilian doctors at the University. Each airman was dissected whilst he was alive on a table that was usually used by medical students to dissect corpses. 'There was no debate among the doctors about whether to do the operations,' recalled Dr. Toshio Tono, who, as a young medical assistant took part in the vivisections in 1945. 'That is what made it so strange,'[11] he said. Tono was so disgusted by what he had witnessed that he published an explosive book on the subject in Japan in the 1980s, against the wishes of his wartime colleagues. It was especially embarrassing as many of them still occupied senior teaching and research positions at the University.

The Americans suffered terribly as the 'operations' were conducted without the benefit of anaesthetics. Stomachs and hearts were opened up, and a study was made about survival with part of the liver missing. Even a portion of the brain of one flyer was excised in order to test a technique for treating epilepsy. Sergeant Teddy Ponczha, the first POW to be experimented upon, was used for a second experiment where his blood was removed and replaced with seawater 'to see if it would work as a substitute for the saline solution normally used as a blood volumizer in medical treatments.'[12] It did not, and Ponczha died in agony. On 17 May 1945, two Americans were experimented upon; on 22 May a further two; on 25 May, a single POW, and on 2 June, three men. On 3 June the liver from the last victim was removed and preserved in preparation for a party that evening in the Officer's Hospital. According to witnesses, the liver was chargrilled and seasoned with soy sauce before being served as an appetizer to the assembled military and civilian guests.

The remains of the American airmen were preserved in the Anatomy Department of Kyushu Imperial University inside glass jars so that students could study them. After the Japanese surrender, and naturally in fear of prosecution for war crimes, the guilty doctors ordered the remains to be disposed of and all records of the experiments destroyed. Stories were quickly concocted to conceal the truth about what had happened to the eight Americans. But, inevitably, news leaked out and soon the American occupation authorities got wind of the story. The Japanese initially stated the airmen had perished during an air raid, but then they changed their story to suggest that the Americans had been conveniently incinerated during the atomic bombing of Hiroshima on 6 August 1945. An investigation by US Military Intelligence and a wave of arrests followed, with a war crimes trial convened in Yokohama in March 1948. One of the surgeons who had vivisected the prisoners, Dr. Fumio Ishiyama, the Chief of Surgery at Kyushu University, committed suicide in jail before he stood trial, indicating his guilt. Eventually, thirty Japanese, some military and some civilian medical personnel, stood trial over the deaths of the eight Americans in Fukuoka. Twenty-three were found guilty and sentenced. Five were sentenced to death by hanging, four to life imprisonment, and the remaining fourteen to shorter periods of detention. However, in the spirit of détente with Japan because the nation had become a very useful ally for the United States during the early phase of the Cold War – particularly during the Korean War – all of the convicted were set free by 1958. None of those sentenced to hang ever did. The whole incident was gradually and effectively written out of history. Kyushu University was certainly very keen to expunge references to the 1945 atrocity from its official history – the 1992 edition of that weighty 700-page tome only includes one page concerning the vivisection experiments. It was only through the efforts of Dr. Tono, who published his damning book about the experiments, that this dark chapter in the history of a venerable academic institution has become more widely known. Today, a small memorial exists to the airmen where their B-29 fell to earth, alongside a similar memorial to the Japanese pilot who rammed his fighter into the big American bomber and killed himself in the process. That is at least some progress towards coming to terms with the horrific deeds of the past.

* * *

At the Mukden Camp the assembled POWs were treated to a display of viciousness by their guards on 6 August 1945. None of the prisoners realised the significance of the date as the guards beat and humiliated them. Word had just reached the Japanese camp authorities that the Americans had dropped a bomb of such awesome power on the city of Hiroshima the metropolis had been virtually wiped off the face of the earth. The Japanese were under no illusions about the outcome of the war, especially when the Soviets launched their invasion two days later.

On 16 or 17 August a four-man OSS team parachuted into Mukden Camp. The team consisted of Major Hennessey, Major Robert Lamar, a military doctor, Sergeant Edward Starz and Corporal Hal Leith. Jumping alongside the OSS men was army interpreter Sergeant Fumio Kido and a representative of the Chinese Nationalist Army. Major Hennessey and his men took control of the camp from the Japanese, and many of the POW officers took on new responsibilities in running the liberated camp until help arrived. The OSS team was very lucky to survive, for when they jumped the Japanese were ignorant of the fact that the war was over. They thought that the six men were Soviet paratroopers who were trying to take over the nearby military airfield. 'On landing they were seized, beaten up, and nearly executed before they could induce the Japanese to look at their credentials, as the Japanese military knew nothing of the capitulation. They did succeed just in time, and were brought to camp,'[13] recalled Major Peaty.

On 18 August a B-29 roared over the camp and dropped leaflets announcing that Japan had surrendered and the war was at long last finally over. The following day T-34 tanks of the Soviet 6th Guards Tank Army, commanded by Major-General Pritula, nosed into Mukden city. The POWs held a church service of thanksgiving and remembrance that finally their salvation had arrived, and they had been delivered from the hell of imprisonment. On 20 August the camp itself was liberated for the second time, this time by a Soviet officer who announced to the assembled POWs that the victorious Red Army had liberated them. General Pritula and many of the Soviet officers worked hard to alleviate some of the suffering of the POWs in those first few days of freedom, and organised the evacuations of the prisoners in concert with the Allied military authorities in Free China. Pritula and several Soviet officers were recommended for American decorations.

For the Japanese guards at Mukden Camp came the moment of truth. Would their abuse and humiliation of the prisoners be

Precedents and Paper Trails

returned in kind? 'At about 7pm a small party of Russian officers arrived and announced that we are now "Svobodo" – free,' recalled Peaty. 'Later in the evening the Japanese guard were disarmed on the parade ground, and headed by their Colonel, marched in single file right around, guarded by us, now wearing their equipment and armed with their weapons, and escorted into their own guardhouse in front of every man in the camp.' Peaty, who spoke Russian, recalled the attitude of the Red Army officers to the Japanese prisoners. 'The Russian officer in charge said "Here they are – do what you like with them, cut their throats or shoot them, it is all the same to me", but this was translated diplomatically as "He says he hands them over to you".'[14] The American and British officers who were now in command of the camp did not take the Soviet officer up on his offer, and instead the Japanese were later turned over as prisoners-of-war to the Chinese Nationalists.

The evacuation of the sickest POWs begun almost at once. On 21 August an American B-24 Liberator left with eighteen POWs who were in urgent need of medical assistance. On 24 August a further twenty-nine were sent out by air, followed by thirty-six of the most senior Allied officers, including Generals Wainwright and Percival, on 27 August. The air evacuation continued until 7 September 1945. Some fighting occurred around the camp between the surrendered Japanese and Chinese guerillas. 'Last night there was a considerable amount of rifle-fire in the vicinity,' wrote Major Peaty, 'and this morning about fifty Japanese were trying to get into camp for protection from the Chinese. We had to put twenty extra men on guard.'[15]

Most of the prisoners were evacuated by trains organised by the Red Army who worked in cooperation with a special nineteen-man US Army group who arrived by plane from Kunming on 29 August. Led by Lieutenant-Colonel James F. Donovan, POW Recovery Team 1 processed out the former prisoners. They dealt with paperwork, issued new clothing, conducted medical evaluations, and identified and exhumed the bodies of POWs who had died at the camp so that their remains could be repatriated. They also brought with them a film projector, and the entertainment-starved former POWs were very grateful. In the meantime, the Americans began sending in supplies. On 29 September 'Four

B.29's arrived in the late afternoon and dropped about 120 parachute loads of supplies'[16], wrote Major Peaty.

Between 10 and 11 September the remaining former POWs at Mukden Camp left by train. A total of 752 left on the 10th, all bound for the port of Darien. Ships were waiting to take them across the Pacific to the United States. The British former prisoners would then cross America by train before shipment across the Atlantic and home. Unfortunately, even though the war was over, men continued to die. Ten former Mukden POWs perished at sea when they were washed overboard from the destroyer USS *Colbert* in a typhoon off Okinawa. Another former POW was killed when the *Colbert* struck a Japanese mine. Major Peaty stepped off a ship in England on 31 October 1945. 'Arrived at Southampton,' he wrote, 'and was both surprised and delighted to find my wife and children at the foot of the gangway as I stepped off.' His last entry in his diary summed up everything: '1.11.45. Home – at last!'[17]

On 19 September 1945 POW Recovery Team 1 closed down Mukden Camp and returned by air to Kunming. The camp stood silent with only the wind stirring the dust of the parade square and lifting the dirty and torn curtains that the prisoners had erected over the windows of their huts. The graveyard was now pockmarked with freshly-dug holes where the Americans had disinterred the hundreds of men who had died of disease. Where once Japanese guards had patrolled with grim expressions and heavy sticks, now only a stray dog picked among the rubbish left behind. The prisoners may have gone, but each of them took this place with them and carried it like an unwanted weight for the rest of their lives. Many would never be free of it, and more than a few would return as old men trying to find answers for all of the things that had happened to them in the camp, and to remember all of their friends and comrades who had had their young lives terminated so abruptly and unnecessarily. The Mukden Camp had been the defining event in most of their lives.

Chapter 8

Flamingo

Secure immediately all Japanese documents and dossiers, and other information useful to the United States government.

Order to the OSS, Manchuria, 13 August 1945

Thompson submachine guns were carefully disassembled and cleaned on the floor of the hut where the American soldiers were waiting for the order to depart. Dressed in olive drab jumpsuits and webbing, each carried a Colt .45 automatic in a brown leather chest holster. They were determined-looking young men with a clear mission directive. Their shoulder patches displayed an oval badge with a golden spearhead against a black background, the insignia of the Office of Strategic Services (OSS). Outside on the grass of the small airfield stood a Dakota transport plane, ready for the off. Engineers were tinkering with the plane while the OSS men nervously smoked cigarettes and listened to the hum of insects through the open windows of the hut. It was a waiting game. Everyone knew that the Japanese were about to surrender and timing was all-essential. If they dropped too early they risked being fired on by the Japanese, but if they landed too late perhaps all the planning would have been for nothing and all they would find would be fires and destruction at the target. Their mission was one of the most important remaining housekeeping duties to perform for America, Operation 'Flamingo'.

Rumours have abounded for years suggesting that some Allied prisoners-of-war may have been taken by the Japanese to the main Unit 731 research facility at Pingfan and used in horrific and terminal human experiments. Hints of Allied POWs who ended up inside the hell of Unit 731 as test subjects have surfaced many times over the past six decades. One former Unit 731 medic, Takeo Wano, said he once saw a six-foot-high glass jar in which a Caucasian man was pickled in formaldehyde. The man had been cut into two pieces, vertically. Specimens like these ominously abounded at the facility.

Another Japanese Unit 731 veteran, who remained anonymous when interviewed in 1995, said he saw specimen jars containing human internal organs, all neatly catalogued. 'I saw labels saying "American", "English" and "Frenchman," but most were Chinese, Koreans and Mongolians,' he recalled. 'Those labeled as American were just body parts, like hands or feet, and some were sent in by other military units.'[1] Some of these 'specimens' may have come from the autopsies that were performed at the Mukden Camp. Two other former Unit 731 personnel, who spoke anonymously at a historical convention held in Morioka City, Japan, in July 1994, had previously related eerily similar stories. The first was a former Youth Corps member. He had been recruited into a Naval Youth Corps unit in Morioka in 1937 and then sent for training at the Army Medical College in Tokyo. By July 1939 he was serving in Unit 731 in Manchuria as part of a team that was researching bacterial propagation. Later in the war he was attached to the National Hygiene Laboratory in Tokyo, where one of his jobs was delivering tins of 16mm film shot at Unit 731 by car to officials of the Imperial Household Agency, the civil servants who ran the Imperial Palace, presumably to be viewed by Emperor Hirohito. 'I preserved a lot of human lab specimens in Formalin,' said the witness in 1995. 'Some were heads, others were arms, legs, internal organs, and some were entire bodies. There were large numbers of these jars lined up, even specimens of children and babies. When I first went into that room I felt sick and couldn't eat for days. But I soon got used to it.' The witness provided some further evidence of what the specimens consisted of. 'Specimens of entire bodies were labeled and identified by nationality, age, sex, and the date and time of death. Names were not identified. There were Chinese, Russians, Koreans, and also Americans, Britons, and Frenchmen. Specimens could have been dissected at this unit or sent in from other subunits; I couldn't tell.'[2] Although it is possible to explain where some of the body parts and organs held at Unit 731 came from, we cannot explain the presence of whole bodies that were labelled 'American' or 'British'. For example, no British prisoners died at the Mukden Camp until very late in the war. Perhaps these 'specimens' came from much further afield, specifically the Shinagawa POW Hospital in Japan, or some similar institution. However, we cannot rule out that these men were killed *inside* Unit 731 at Pingfan, as rumours have persisted this was indeed the case.

The second Japanese witness, who also remained anonymous, was a hygiene specialist who, in March 1941, had been transferred to the main Unit 731 research facility at Pingfan. He admitted witnessing many experiments conducted upon Chinese prisoners. At Unit 731 in June 1941 he saw inside a building that was located close to the officers' married quarters. 'I noticed, farther inside at a wide space in the corridor, there was a human specimen in a jar,' he said in 1994. 'The jar was the size of a person, and what looked like a young Russian soldier was preserved inside in liquid. His body was cut in half, lengthwise. I realised later that it was a White Russian.'[3] The witness also said there were other human-sized glass jars stacked alongside the one containing the Russian body, but they were covered and he never saw the contents. Later that night the witness was beaten by a Japanese officer for having looked at what was expressly forbidden. This occurred before the Japanese attack on the United States in December 1941, but nonetheless, it demonstrates that physicians at Unit 731 were already preserving the corpses of Caucasian prisoners murdered by them as early as March 1941 – and as demonstrated by the other two witnesses whose testimonies have already been outlined, the bodies of American, British and French men were seen preserved in an identical manner later in the war.

Other Japanese witnesses have confirmed there were most certainly Caucasian prisoners held at Pingfan until the very last weeks of the war, but the only nationality positively determined is Russian. Shiro Ishii's personal driver, Sadao Koshi, who was also employed at Unit 731, driving the truck that took prisoners to the facility's gas chamber, recalled the treatment of a group of Russian prisoners shipped in to Pingfan towards the end of the war. 'Around June 1945, we knew that things were coming to an end,' said Koshi. 'About that time, one day a truckload of about forty Russians came in. There were a lot of *maruta* already in hand, and there could be no need for them. So, the Russians were told that there was an epidemic in the region, and that they should get off the truck to get preventive injections. Then they were injected with potassium cyanide. The men administering the injections rubbed the arms of the Russians with alcohol first. If you're going to kill someone, there's no need to disinfect the injection arm; that was just to conceal the real intention.' Koshi recalled the ease with which the Russians were murdered. 'It only took a small amount [of cyanide], and even those big Russians fell back as soon as the injection was given. They didn't even make a sound – they just dropped.'[4]

Unit 731 veterans have recalled that other Caucasian nationalities, besides Russians, were also present at Pingfan during the war. Another Japanese who stood trial at Khabarovsk in 1949, Kiyohito Morishita, stated in court: '[The] Soviets and Americans can be distinguished in appearance. Among the *maruta* I saw Americans or British. I also heard some *marutas* speaking English to each other.'[5] Morishita was referring to the Unit 731 facility at Pingfan where he worked, and not to the Mukden Camp. His testimony suggests that Allied POWs were taken from Mukden to Pingfan, experimented on and then killed. If they had not come from Mukden, then these prisoners may easily have come from other camps within the Japanese Empire, for with hundreds of thousands of Allied soldiers under their control, the Japanese were certainly not short of possible test subjects.

The problem for historians has been trying to find evidence that prisoners were shipped out of Mukden Camp to Unit 731. All that can be established, from the available documentary evidence, is that around two hundred prisoners were removed from the camp, and that at the time, the witnesses to this movement did not know where the men were being taken to. The inmates at Mukden did not see them again, leading some to assert foul play on the part of the Japanese. Australian Army doctor Captain R.J. Brennan recorded in his secret diary an incident where 150 American prisoners were force marched out of Mukden Camp and never seen again. Major Robert Peaty also recorded the same event. As previously noted, the Japanese removed 150 POWs from the camp on 24 May 1944 and shipped them to Japan to work in the Mitsubishi-owned mine at Kamisha. In June 1944 a further fifty American POWs were sent to Kamisha as punishment for sabotaging the factories at Mukden. The prisoners were shipped to Japan to work as slave labourers and many of them were liberated at the end of the war. They were not sent to Pingfan and can be discounted from any investigation.

In 1994 a document surfaced at the US National Archives in Washington D.C. which has provided another clue towards answering the question of whether Allied POWs were experimented upon at Pingfan. The document, dated 13 August 1945, is a series of orders issued by the Office of Strategic Services (OSS), related to the launching of an operation that was codenamed 'Flamingo'.

The OSS was President Roosevelt's response to Churchill's creation of the Special Operations Executive (SOE). Established by Presidential Order in June 1942, OSS teams played a major role in the Far East, particularly with the training of Nationalist Chinese forces in China and Burma, the recruitment and training of indigenous tribesmen in the Burmese highlands, and the arming and training of communist revolutionaries in China and French Indochina. China was considered an American intelligence responsibility during the war, whereas the British dealt with Southeast Asia. SOE's local unit was known as Force 136 and operated in close cooperation with the Australians. OSS Detachment 404 was based at Admiral Lord Mountbatten's Southeast Asia Command Headquarters at Kandy in Ceylon, and mounted joint operations with the British, while there were four other OSS detachments elsewhere in Asia that operated independently.[6]

It appears from the document that US military intelligence were aware the Japanese were conducting biological weapons research in Manchuria, and that this involved human experimentation at a facility near the city of Harbin. It is also clear the Americans suspected that Allied POWs were some of the victims of these experiments. A lightly armed fifteen-man OSS team was ordered to liberate American and Allied prisoners-of-war by flying into the Harbin area 'on a moment's notice on V-J day'.[7] The team was instructed 'to immediately contact all Allied POW Camps' in the area, to 'notify headquarters of the number, condition, etc. of the prisoners in the concentration camps', and 'to render any medical assistance necessary and feasible.'[8] The only problem with this plan was that the nearest concentration of Allied POWs was over three hundred miles away in Mukden, and therefore this part of the order did not make sense. Was 'Flamingo' a case of faulty intelligence, or did the Americans know something about Pingfan that has hitherto never been revealed to the public?

The complexity of launching an operation into Occupied China, with the nearest American forces in the Philippines and Nationalist China, attests to this not being a case of faulty intelligence. In fact, rescue efforts were underway all across Asia, with both OSS and British SOE teams ready to parachute in to Japanese POW camps which had already been identified by covert observation and co-operation with indigenous resistance networks, and this was to occur the moment the Emperor surrendered. The fear was that the Japanese, even in defeat, would slaughter their prisoners to prevent their liberation. This Allied fear was grounded in fact, as the Japanese military high command had promulgated such orders to all POW camp commandants the previous year.

It had been official Japanese policy since 1 August 1944 that prisoners would not be left behind to be liberated by the advancing Allies. The War Ministry in Tokyo had issued clear instructions to Japanese occupation forces across Asia to 'prevent the prisoners of war from falling into the enemy's hands.'[9] The order read in part: 'Under the present situation if there were a mere explosion or fire a shelter for the time being could be had in nearby buildings such as the school, a warehouse, or the like. However, at such time as the situation became urgent and it be extremely important, the POWs will be concentrated and confined in their present location and under heavy guard the preparation for the final disposition will be made.'[10] The War Ministry had then further instructed that commanders were well within their rights to kill all of their prisoners without fear of censure or punishment. It clearly set out the conditions for such an action:

'Although the basic aim is to act under superior orders, Individual disposition may be made in the following circumstances: (a) When an uprising of large numbers cannot be suppressed without the use of firearms; (b) When escapees from the camp may turn into a hostile Fighting force.' The final part of the order detailed suggested methods for disposing of the prisoners: '(a) Whether they are destroyed individually or in groups, or however it is done, with mass bombing, poisonous smoke, poisons, drowning, decapitation, or what, dispose of them as the situation dictates.'[11]

Flamingo

Sadayoshi Nakanishi, Acting Director of the Prisoner of War Information Bureau in Tokyo, had in his possession when he was captured after the war, a document that reiterated the earlier orders referred to above. Dated 11 March 1945, it stated: 'Prisoners of War must be prevented *by all possible means* [author's italics] from falling into enemy hands.'[12] It also reiterated earlier orders that changing the location of prisoner-of-war camps ahead of the advancing Allies was necessary to preserve the prisoners as slave labour for as long as possible, but that prisoners could be released 'In the event of an enemy attack which leaves no alternative ...'[13]

This was obviously a contradictory stance, but typical of Japanese bureaucratic confusion present throughout the prison camp system. Perhaps the orders were left deliberately vague and contradictory so that local commanders could interpret them as they saw fit in the fluid circumstances that they found themselves in.

The surviving documentary evidence does strongly suggest that local Japanese commanders were under specific orders to keep Allied prisoners and internees alive for as long as possible for use as labour, but if faced with imminent defeat and the liberation of those prisoners by advancing Allied forces, the commanders were ordered to kill them by any means at hand.

Orders were even issued which instructed 'brutal guards and commanders to flee.' The rationale behind this order, issued on 20 August 1945, five days *after* the Japanese surrender, was simple. 'Personnel who mistreated prisoners of war and internees or who are held in extremely bad sentiment by them are permitted to take care of it by immediately transferring or by fleeing without trace.'[14] Finally, orders were also issued to destroy incriminating documents and files ahead of the arrival of Allied forces. This order was somewhat superfluous as many local Japanese commanders had already been doing this in the last days of the war, including Shiro Ishii at Pingfan. It read: 'Documents which would be unfavorable for us in the hands of the enemy are to be treated in the same way as secret documents and destroyed when finished with.'[15]

The seizure of documents was of especially high priority to the OSS team that would be launched by Operation Flamingo into Manchuria. The Flamingo orders perhaps reveal how much the Americans knew about Unit 731. The 13 August 1945 order instructed the team to 'secure immediately all Japanese documents and dossiers, and other information useful to the United States government.'[16] From this sentence we can see that US military intelligence was fully appraised of the significance of the work that Shiro Ishii and his colleagues were conducting at Pingfan. None of the other OSS 'humanitarian' rescue teams that were dropped into Occupied Asia in August 1945 had been issued orders other than to prevent the Japanese guards from murdering Allied POWs, and to begin to organise the POWs' medical stabilisation and evacuation. It might be argued, based upon the language of the Operation Flamingo orders, that securing the biological warfare data at Pingfan was *the* priority, and rescuing any Allied POWs was a secondary priority. It is also interesting to note that all other POW rescue units parachuted into camps by the Americans and British generally consisted of only four or five lightly-armed officers and men. Flamingo called for the immediate deployment of *fifteen* military intelligence operatives. The whole issue of Allied POWs being held at Pingfan appears disingenuous and designed as a 'cover story' for the real OSS mission. We might interpret the Flamingo orders as follows: Perhaps OSS knew that no Allied POWs were actually held at Pingfan and the section of the operational orders that instructed its operatives to secure prisoners-of-war was simply a ruse, giving the Americans a pretext to secure Pingfan ahead of the advancing Soviet Red Army that had invaded Manchuria on 8 August 1945. The Soviets were advancing south rapidly against a weakened Japanese Kwantung Army and would shortly capture the Unit 731 facility at Pingfan. Because the evidence of live Allied POWs being held at Pingfan is so sketchy and incomplete, it is impossible to give a definitive answer regarding the real intentions of the Flamingo planners.

The debate over Operation Flamingo has to remain academic as events swiftly overtook the plans of the OSS. The sudden Japanese surrender on 15 August 1945, only two days after the orders had been drafted for Flamingo, severely wrong-footed the Americans. Events in Manchuria had also passed the stage where the Americans could have intervened. Operation 'Autumn Storm', the vast Soviet offensive into Manchuria and Korea, had made rapid progress since its launch on 8 August and on V-J Day the Red Army was in control of a partially-ruined Pingfan facility. One of Ishii's final acts before he escaped with most of his staff and their precious records and dossiers, was to order Unit 731 destroyed. The job was botched and, as we will see, the Soviets seized the facility, along with many of its staff. Mukden Camp had also been liberated by a Soviet armoured spearhead, the weakened Japanese Kwantung Army proving no match for hardened Soviet troops who had been fighting through the ruins of Berlin only three months before. The Soviets committed widespread atrocities against captured Japanese, and sought to swiftly establish communist puppet regimes behind them. They were also preparing to invade Japan from the north, and the realisation that most of the nation's defences were concentrated on the southern island of Kyushu and expecting to repel a huge American and British assault, meant that the country would have quickly fallen under Stalin's direct rule. As the Japanese were only fighting on so ferociously in order to preserve the position of the Emperor in any postwar state, it was better to surrender quickly to the democratic Western Allies than see their entire culture subsumed under Moscow's iron rule. The effect of the two atomic bombings of Japanese cities really played a minor part in deciding the timing of the Japanese surrender. Fear of the Soviets, and of communism, was a far more compelling reason to stop fighting.

As we will see later, the Americans were already considering how they could lay their hands on the scientists and their all-important biological warfare data which had slipped out from under the noses of the Soviets when Pingfan had been abandoned in flames. Flamingo indicates that the OSS and the American government were determined to snatch Ishii and his research results to use in the coming Cold War with the Soviet Union. The question of whether or not American and Allied POWs formed a part of those research results was not important to Washington, as the practical expediencies of preparing for the coming ideological showdown with Moscow took precedence over all other considerations. It would certainly explain why so many documents from the era that would probably settle the question of Allied POW experiments remain outside of the public domain, making the 1956 memorandum to FBI Director J. Edgar Hoover written on the subject, appear persuasive evidence of a high-level cover-up.

Chapter 9

Reaping the Whirlwind

> *Such information could not be obtained in our own laboratories because of scruples attached to human experimentation.*
>
> Dr. Edwin Hill, Camp Detrick biological warfare centre, December 1947

The destruction and abandonment of the main Unit 731 facility at Pingfan was the greatest blow to American ambitions. As we have seen, the Americans had been about to launch an OSS team to retrieve valuable documentation from the facility when the war had abruptly ended. It is worth looking at how the Soviet Union became an important player in the last stages of the war in Asia, and in the story of Unit 731.

The Soviets came fresh from the vicious ideological war with Nazi Germany. They were skilled and ruthless fighters who cared little for their own casualties, and were not in the business of showing their enemies much in the way of mercy either. At the 1945 Yalta Conference convened between Prime Minister Winston Churchill, President Harry S. Truman and Premier Josef Stalin, the Soviets had listened to Allied pleas to terminate the Soviet-Japan Non-Aggression Pact they had signed in 1941. The Pact had been extremely useful during the war with Germany, for it had maintained an uneasy peace between the two armies staring at each other across the Manchurian-Mongolian border north of China. Stalin made a promise to join the Pacific War against Japan three months after Germany surrendered. The Germans surrendered on 8 May 1945 and, true to his word, Operation

'August Storm', the Soviet invasion of Manchuria, was unleashed on 8 August 1945.

Marshal Aleksandr Vasilevsky led a massive invasion force of over one-and-a-half million Red Army troops and 3,704 tanks against the much-depleted Kwantung Army. The Japanese force, under the command of General Otsuzo Yamada, could field just over one million men in Manchuria and about one thousand tanks, but most of its best units had already been hived off earlier in the war to fight the Americans in the Pacific and Anglo-Indian forces in Burma, and its tanks were inferior in every way to the fabulous Soviet T-34. One of the limiting factors of the Japanese strategy in the Pacific had been the requirement to station a very large force on the Mongolian border to deter any Soviet ambitions in northern China. As the war progressed, and with no indications that Stalin would break his non-aggression agreement with Japan, the best commanders, units and equipment had been stripped from the Kwantung Army and shipped elsewhere to shore up Japanese defences.

The Red Army had absorbed all of the hard and costly lessons it had learned fighting the Germans in European Russia and Eastern Europe, and compared with the Japanese, their tactics were superior, their officers better trained, and their tanks out-classed anything the Japanese could field. In the air, the Red Army Air Force quickly established air superiority over Manchuria. The Japanese fought with their usual suicidal bravery, but it was all to no avail, as Soviet armoured columns quickly burst through the Japanese lines and advanced south into Manchuria with little to stop them. At the same time, the Soviets launched amphibious invasions of northern Korea, southern Sakhalin, and the Kurile Islands. On 14 August 1945 Japan surrendered unconditionally and the Soviet advance shuddered to a halt just short of the Korean border.

The Japanese historian Tsuyoshi Hasegawa in *Racing the Enemy: Stalin, Truman, and the Surrender of Japan*, has suggested that the American atomic bombings of Hiroshima and Nagasaki had little effect on the Japanese will to fight on, but that Operation 'Autumn Storm' was *the* event that forced the Japanese government to surrender quickly. The Soviet advance had been so rapid that their next target was clearly an amphibious assault on Hokkaido in the north of Japan. Stalin would have made this assault far in advance of the planned American and British invasion of Kyushu in the south that was not due to begin until December 1945, and most of the strongest Japanese forces, including nearly all-remaining combat aircraft, were in the south preparing to fend off the Anglo-American invasion. The north of Japan was effectively wide open, and the awful prospect of the Soviets overrunning most of Japan in short order became a reality. If they had, Emperor Hirohito would undoubtedly have been placed on trial as a war criminal and Japan would have quickly been absorbed as a communist satellite state of the Soviet Union, as was happening at the time throughout all of Eastern Europe. Such a fate was too awful for the Japanese leaders to contemplate, and so ending the war quickly became a priority. Although some elements inside the Japanese military attempted to stage a coup in Tokyo to prevent news of the surrender from being broadcast to the troops, this was quickly crushed and an unconditional capitulation announced.

Tens of thousands were killed on both sides during 'Autumn Storm', and the Soviets and Japanese have never agreed upon the exact casualty figures. As the Soviet juggernaut cleaved through the weakened Japanese Kwantung Army like a hot knife, Stalin's Red Army began liberating the victims of the Japanese prison camp system, finding scenes of suffering and deprivation as great as those that they had witnessed in the Nazi concentration and extermination camps they had liberated on their way to Berlin six months before. But with liberation came problems. The Soviets descended like a latter-day Mongol horde, killing, raping, looting and pillaging, the Japanese absolutely powerless to stop them.

Lieutenant General Ishii ordered the scientists and doctors at Unit 731 to be evacuated to Japan before the Red Army arrived at Pingfan. He also ordered the destruction of the facility in an attempt to cover-up the extent of the crimes that had been committed by the men under his command. A special unit of *Kempeitai* soldiers was detailed for this important task, but it was largely a botched attempt as the place was too well constructed and withstood the effects of localised demolitions.

The efficient South Manchurian Railway was the quickest route out of the region for the large Unit 731 staff and their families, and a special train was laid on by the Japanese military that took the personnel from Pingfan and Harbin south through Korea, managing to stay just ahead of the Soviets. From Korea it was a short journey by ship to Japan, whence another special train took the scientists and their families north through the city of Kanazawa where some of the Unit's members disembarked and took refuge in the local Nome Shrine. The train then continued on into Niigata Prefecture where the passengers split up and went their separate ways back into Japanese society hoping to avoid detection. During the first part of the escape from Manchuria, Ishii had accompanied his staff on the train. While they went by ship to Japan, he boarded a special aircraft with his extensive files and films. Before taking to the air Ishii warned his colleagues in no uncertain terms. He told them never to take jobs in public offices, never to contact each other, and to take the secret of Unit 731 with them to their graves. Ishii implied that anyone who refused to honour this code of silence would be tracked down in Japan and punished. Considering Ishii's power and influence among the Japanese elite, it was not an idle threat, and his colleagues knew how ruthless he could be.

Although most of the scientists managed to escape from Manchuria, as mentioned the small number of *Kempeitai* troops who had been left behind and tasked with destroying the facility at Pingfan, were largely unsuccessful because the buildings had been so well constructed before the war, and there was insufficient time remaining to make a thorough job of it. Important evidence was thus left intact, and it did not take long for the Soviets, and later the Chinese, to figure out what those red brick buildings had been used for. At some of the other Unit 731 sites even less was done to conceal their secret use; at Unit 1644 in Nanjing the Japanese stationed there simply cleared off with their records and specimens in a fleet of army trucks for the nearest airport, abandoning the building to the Chinese. Today, it serves as a hospital in the city with the vast majority of the patients who pass through its doors having no idea of the building's horrific wartime history. This apathy towards the horrors of the past is quite a common feature of modern China, for many buildings used by the Japanese for the most inhumane of reasons continue to be used without the least qualms. For example, in Shanghai a building called Bridge House, close to the famous Bund, which served from 1937 to 1945 as the main torture and murder centre for the *Kempeitai* military police, is today an apartment building crammed with local families.

Shiro Ishii, and his fellow scientists and researchers, went to great lengths to save the enormous wealth of data they had obtained from their twenty-year human experimentation programme in Manchuria and elsewhere. With the war now lost, that data was to become their greatest bargaining chip. Ishii and the others knew that the Allies were preparing to place some Japanese on trial for war crimes, as they had done to the defeated Germans who had faced justice at Nuremberg, and the Unit 731 veterans were determined that they would not be the ones who would pay the price for their nation's empire building in Asia. Many of them actually believed their activities at Unit 731 had advanced scientific knowledge, regardless of the cruelty and murder that had accompanied their research, and that they were simple doctors and scientists.

For its part the United States, which assumed the occupation of Japan from September 1945 under the control of General Douglas MacArthur, had appointed a well-regarded Columbia University microbiologist named Dr. Murray Sanders to investigate the Japanese biological warfare programme. Commissioned for the duration as a lieutenant colonel in the US Army, during the war Sanders was attached to Camp Detrick, America's main biological weapons research facility. Somehow, the Japanese knew of Sanders imminent arrival aboard the USS *Sturgess* at Yokohama in September 1945 and they dispatched a senior Unit 731 scientist to meet him on the quayside, effectively reaching out before the Americans began to search for them.

Sanders had never heard of the designation 'Unit 731', so he was not initially suspicious of the polite Japanese man who was holding his photograph and carefully scanning the faces of the uniformed passengers as they disembarked down the gangplank from the ship. The Japanese man standing on the quayside was none other than Lieutenant-Colonel Dr. Ryoichi Naito, a close confidante of Shiro Ishii who, amongst other posts, had been an important member of the Tokyo laboratory of Unit 731. He cleverly introduced himself as Sander's interpreter. Colonel Sanders was soon ensconced in an office in Tokyo and beginning the task of finding and interviewing Japan's biological warfare elite, with one of their most senior men unwittingly sitting by his side. Every evening Dr. Naito would disappear to have secret meetings at various Japanese military headquarters around the city, keeping the Unit 731 people fully abreast of the developing American investigation.

Taking his instructions from higher authorities, Dr. Naito carefully fed Sanders information about Japan's biological weapons programme and at the same time kept the Japanese side fully informed of Sanders' interrogations of suspects. From this pivotal position, Naito effectively stymied Sanders' investigation, leading to considerable exasperation on the American side. Realising he was being 'played', Sanders decided to up the ante with the Japanese by threatening them with the one thing that they most feared. He told Naito bluntly that unless things changed rapidly he would have no choice but to invite the Soviets to take part in the investigation. 'I said that because the Japanese exhibited a deadly fear of the Communists, and they didn't want them messing around,' recalled Colonel Sanders. 'He [Naito] appeared the next morning with a manuscript which contained startling material. It was fundamentally dynamite. The manuscript said, in essence, that the Japanese were involved in biological warfare.'[1]

A copy of the manuscript was passed to the British who scrutinised it very carefully. The Inter-Service Sub-Committee on Biological Warfare called it a general summary of Japanese biological warfare activities with some information on the policy of the Japanese military authorities. 'No documents or experimental protocols were available to the [American] interrogators, and the drawings included in the report were based on sketches supplied by the Japanese to Colonel Sanders,'[2] noted the British. The British, like the Americans, were fully aware of the existence of a large experimental facility at Pingfan in Manchuria, and that it had been in operation for eight years, but scientists from Britain's chemical and biological warfare centre at Porton Down in Wiltshire who examined the American material did not yet understand the extent of the Japanese biological warfare programme. 'Despite all this work, the report had practically no technical information of value, and what little there was suggests the work was carried out in a strangely crude and amateurish manner,'[3] was the blunt British assessment.

Sanders took the manuscript to General MacArthur, who as the military governor of Japan, was the most powerful man in the country. Accompanying the manuscript was an organisational chart for Unit 731. It included the names of medical and military detachments who had produced germs and used animals for biological warfare research, as well as their administrative departments. The chart showed Emperor Hirohito at the top, and then the chain of command passing down through the Imperial General Staff in Tokyo, the Bureau of Medical Affairs, and the headquarters of the Kwantung Army, China Expeditionary Force (which occupied Central China), and the Southern Army (covering South China, Indochina, Malaya, and the Netherlands East Indies). Importantly, none of the documents that were initially handed to Sanders had made any mention of human experimentation. At this stage the Japanese idea was to whet Allied appetites rather than serve a main course. General MacArthur made his decision regarding the Unit 731 personnel without all of the facts regarding the extent of Japanese criminality in front of him, but when it became obvious that Dr. Ishii and his men had killed thousands of people as a bi-product of their research, such an ethical consideration did not ultimately weigh heavily upon the Americans, or indeed with their British allies.

General MacArthur immediately seized on the importance of the information contained within the documents brought to him by Sanders. The potential data that could come from Naito and his colleagues was almost incalculable and incredibly valuable to the United States. Most importantly, America wanted that information, wrote MacArthur, 'on an exclusive basis.'[4] But in order to obtain the information they desired, the Americans were left with no choice but to strike a deal with the Japanese sources. As MacArthur pointed out to Sanders, the United States could not use coercion to obtain the desired information, and so an ultimately regrettable, though understandable, decision was reached. Sanders was instructed to offer Naito and his friends immunity from prosecution at the forthcoming Tokyo Trials in return for their full cooperation in providing the United States with all available research into biological weapons. The decision was certainly highly immoral once the Americans were fully appraised of the facts of Unit 731's wartime activities, but the exigencies of the coming Cold War meant that the Americans could abandon their higher-minded humanitarian principles for the sake of their national security without many objections being raised in government circles.

American investigators interrogated seven of the most senior Japanese military officers who could have known in detail about the goings-on at Unit 731, with the important exception at this stage of Shiro Ishii himself. In a report dated 1 November 1945, Sanders paraphrased a meeting with Lieutenant General Kambayashi, Surgeon General to the Imperial Japanese Army, during which Kambayashi 'stated that he personally was opposed to the use of B.W. [biological warfare] on humanitarian and practical grounds.'[5] Even more unbelievable was Kambayashi's next assertion: 'He stated that as far as he knew, no offensive studies on B.W. had been made.' The Japanese Army's most senior doctor 'admitted the possibility that the Kwantung armies had carried out research unknown to the authorities in Tokyo,'[6] a statement that was designed, as we now know, to suggest to the Americans that the horrors of Unit 731 were nothing to do with the army, or the Japanese government, and were instead the work of a 'rogue element' within the military that had operated on the far borders of the Japanese empire. 'The Surgeon General knew of General Ishii but apparently the latter was not popular in Tokyo and was considered a pushing type of officer.'[7] This lie was later fed to the British by the Americans when London became acutely interested in having the Americans share the biological warfare data they had in their possession. 'As far as can be ascertained, the Japanese high command was opposed to the use of B.W.' stated the Chairman of the Inter-Service Sub-Committee on Biological Warfare, Air Marshal Sir Norman Bottomley, in May 1946. 'The high command therefore initiated no work on the subject and apparently knew little of the work that was done, although this was said to be considerable.'[8] The British also knew very little about the Pingfan facility because they were denied access to the Japanese scientists that were being intensively questioned by the Americans in Tokyo. 'The Pingfan institute was said to have been destroyed before it was overrun by the Russian Army,' noted Bottomley. 'Technical determinations of the work carried out at Pingfan are very vague owing to the absence of written records.'[9] It was those written records that General MacArthur and his subordinates were about to access.

Once a deal had been struck, a huge amount of fascinating material landed in the Americans' laps. 'In subsequent meetings, US military interviewers received a flood of information including many autopsy reports of Chinese and Russian vivisection victims, and thousands of slide samples of human tissues and germ warfare pathogens.'[10] The British, although they did not know the full details of the secret deal, nonetheless asked the Americans for more information. In fact, the British asked on several occasions for 'the Americans to make further detailed investigations about this establishment [Pingfan] and that, if possible, records of actual field trials and other work carried out by the Japanese should be secured.'[11] This was precisely what the Americans were doing, but in the process they were deliberately failing to pass on really useful data to the British. It was not in America's best interests to allow even its closest ally an edge in biological weapons research. Instead, the British were initially left with vague reports and summaries which contributed virtually nothing to their own BW research at Porton Down in Wiltshire.

The decision taken by General MacArthur to offer Ishii, Naito, and the others a deal also meant that Unit 731 and its ghastly activities remained a largely unknown organization for far longer than it should have. There would be no justice for the tens of thousands of men, women and children who had been sacrificed by the Japanese on the altar of medical science, and this in fact remains the *status quo*. The American back-stairs deal granted the Japanese war criminals who created and ran Unit 731 blanket immunity from prosecution *in perpetuity*. Whether this was a right decision because American national security demanded biological weapons to potentially fight the Soviet Union in any putative 'World War III' remains very controversial to answer. What is clear is that the suffering and deaths of the people who were sent to Unit 731 was less of a concern to the American government and military than gaining the information and data that had been generated by their murders.

When the issue of whether American and British POWs had been experimented on alongside Chinese and Russian prisoners was first raised, the issue was deftly sidestepped by the American government and subsequently consigned to the realm of fantasy, where the topic currently languishes six-and-a-half decades later. It was one thing to benefit from experiments that had been conducted on foreigners, but quite another to use data gathered from the suffering and deaths of one's own soldiers and those of one's closest ally. That would have been completely reprehensible and have led to all sorts of problems with the press and the general public in both countries. For this reason, it can be surmised that the truth about Unit 731 experiments on Allied POWs at the Mukden Camp will remain classified forever, and the official position of the American and British governments will also remain one of flat denial. This is not to say they were told several times of the likelihood that the Japanese had indeed used Allied POWs, the first warning emerging soon after the Japanese surrender.

The first intimation the Americans had of the possible use by the Japanese of Allied POWs in human experiments came shortly after General MacArthur had offered Dr. Naito and his associates immunity from prosecution. On 6 January 1946 the American armed forces newspaper *Pacific Stars and Stripes* ran a story that had originated with the Japanese Communist Party. It stated boldly that the Japanese had experimented on American POWs. The story named Shiro Ishii as the chief instigator of this programme. The story said Ishii had directed human biological warfare experiments using American and Chinese prisoners at Mukden and Harbin. The *New York Times* picked up and ran this story as well. In response, American investigators pulled Ishii in for questioning in Tokyo on 12 January 1946, but he sensibly denied having experimented on Allied POWs, or Russians, and was believed for the time being.

MacArthur, Supreme Commander of the Allied Powers (SCAP), next received a letter dated 10 February 1946 from a man named Takeshi Kino which alleged there had been experiments on Allied POWs and named three of Ishii's associates as being responsible for having 'dissected many war prisoners of the Allied Forces at the outdoor dissecting ground of Unit 100 Army Corps at Hsingking [now Changchun], Manchuria, at their inspections of the cattle plague.'[12] A letter dated 4 October 1946 was also sent to General MacArthur. It was written by a man named Hiroshi Ueki, and alleged: 'Lieutenant General Shiro Ishii ... executed brutal experiments on many Allied POWs.'[13] In 1947 American Military Intelligence prepared a report on Dr. Ishii's wartime activities, and during the course of this document *twelve* separate allegations were made by twelve different sources that all stated that Ishii and his colleagues had used Allied POWs in human experiments. Later that same year, a further intelligence memorandum noted: 'Legal Section, SCAP, stated in cable No. C53169, dated 7 June 1947, that the Japanese Communist Party alleges that Ishii BW group conducted experiments on captured Americans in Mukden and that simultaneously research on similar lines was conducted in Tokyo and Kyoto.'[14] 'Tokyo' could be a reference to the well-documented biological warfare tests which were conducted on Allied POWs at the Shinagawa POW Hospital located close to the city. In fact, in August 1947 an American government document admitted that 'there is a remote possibility that independent investigations conducted by the Soviets in the Mukden area may have disclosed evidence that American prisoners of war were used for experimental purposes of a BW nature and that they lost their lives as a result of these experiments.'[15]

As we have seen previously, during the course of the Khabarovsk War Crimes Trial in Siberia in 1949, Major Tomio Karasawa, a former section chief at Unit 731, did admit in court that American POWs had been used for biological warfare testing at Mukden. Clearly the Americans put more faith in the Soviet investigation than was subsequently revealed. And, as we have also seen, in 1956 an attempt by the FBI to investigate this matter was terminated after hitting a brick wall of secrecy. The investigating agent wrote to J. Edgar Hoover, stating: '... information of the type in question is closely controlled and regarded as highly sensitive.'

All of this suggests a high-level cover-up. It can be surmised that the American government was determined the truth would be withheld from the public for the simple reason that the Americans had secretly used captured Japanese biological warfare data which had come, in part, from experiments upon, and the deaths of, American citizens. To have fully admitted the truth would have opened the government to a charge of callous disregard of its moral obligations to the victims of Japanese aggression, and to a charge of applying selective justice against those Japanese who were suspected, with good reason, of having committed war crimes. Not far away from where Colonel Sanders and his assistants were busily collecting information from Ishii, Naito and the other Unit 731 scientists, the International Military Tribunal for the Far East, the Japanese equivalent of the Nuremberg Trials in Germany, had opened in May 1946. This was four months *after* Shiro Ishii had first spoken to American investigators.

Chief of the International Prosecution Section (IPS) at the trial, Joseph Keenan, had by May 1946 received reports concerning biological warfare experimentation and the deployment of BW weapons in the field by the Japanese military. However, no action was taken to investigate whether any of the Japanese known to US Army Chemical Corps investigators should have been called to testify in court. The IPS informed the War Department in Washington D.C. that the testimony from Unit 731 officers and from men the Red Army had captured in Manchuria in August 1945, which the Soviet had already recorded, was convincing enough that it 'warrants conclusion that Japanese BW group headed by Ishii did violate rules of land warfare, but this expression of opinion is not a recommendation that group be charged and tried for such.'[16] The United States had no desire to see Unit 731's secrets blurted out in court and they certainly intended to remain the sole beneficiary of that information.

The Soviet's chief prosecutor at the Tokyo trials demanded that representatives of his nation be granted access to Ishii and two of his colleagues so that they might question them in detail. The two Japanese officers whom the Soviets were most keen to speak to were Colonel Kiyoshi Ota, who was responsible for the plague bombing of the Chinese city of Changde in November 1941, and Colonel Hitoshi Kikuchi, another top Unit 731 commander. These officers had been implicated in germ warfare attacks by some of their colleagues who had been captured and interrogated by the Soviets. The Soviet interest in these three men, and Unit 731 more generally, was simple. Moscow wanted to investigate the unit's activities which had, after all, occurred immediately adjacent to Soviet territory. The USSR also had a desire for revenge against the Japanese for their use of biological weapons against Red Army troops and Soviet citizens. Finally, the request was an excellent chance to obtain, in the words of Hal Gold, author of *Unit 731 Testimony*, 'grist for the propaganda mill'.[17]

A formal Soviet request was made to General MacArthur on 9 January 1947. Considering that the Americans were well aware that many of the scientific samples they now held had come from Russian citizens who had been murdered by the Japanese, it was a fair request. Naturally, however, the American intelligence community was not so keen on the idea, feeling that it was important to limit access to the Unit 731 personnel in the hope of benefitting exclusively from their knowledge. Indeed, on 24 January the Joint Chiefs of Staff in Washington D.C. issued an instruction to MacArthur ordering him to make sure that the gruesome human experiments and mass murders that had been committed by Unit 731 staff be kept secret from the American public, and from friendly governments, such as the British government. 'All intelligence information that may be detrimental to the security of the country or possibly detrimental to the friendly countries must be held confidential,' read the Joint Chiefs order, 'the release of which must have prior approval from the Joint Chiefs of Staff and if necessary with the consent of the State-War-Navy-Coordinating Committee (SWNCC).'[18] The SWNCC was a combined military and State Department group based in the American capital that had ultimate responsibility for American occupation policy in Germany and Japan. This policy appears to have been followed, for British documents suggest that London did not understand yet where most of the valuable data had come from. 'Vague accounts have been obtained of the organisation [Unit 731] which were considered and of field trials which were carried out, but there is no indication of any substantial developments or of large scale culturing for offensive purposes,' reported the British. They believed at this stage that the Japanese had been using animals for the testing. 'It is said that in two years work on anthrax, 100 horses and 500 sheep were used in field trials.'[19]

General MacArthur passed on the Soviet request to the Joint Chiefs in Washington D.C. on 7 February 1947. On 21 March the Joint Chiefs told MacArthur to permit the Soviet agents access to Ishii and the two other Japanese officers they had named, but MacArthur was to make sure that his intelligence people instructed the Japanese not to reveal anything important about the biological warfare programme to the Soviets. The Japanese were thus carefully coached, and they happily cooperated as a way of ensuring their continued freedom from prosecution for war crimes. MacArthur even managed to delay the meetings until mid-May 1947 and instructed that American officers had to be in the room with the Soviet interviewer at all times. Whether the Soviets realised that the Unit 731 veterans were simply spouting the American line is not recorded, but it is a safe assumption to state that the NKVD were not stupid, and they must have suspected the American motives, and the Japanese behaviour and responses to their questions.

By this time, Colonel Sanders had returned to the United States. His replacement in Tokyo was Dr. Arvo Thompson, an American microbiologist who had been commissioned as a colonel into the US Army Chemical Corps. Dr. Norbert Fell assisted him in questioning numerous top Unit 731 scientists and researchers during this period, securing a veritable bounty of fascinating data to assist the American biological warfare programme at Camp Detrick. Nineteen Japanese scientists presented Fell with a 200-page report on crop destruction experiments, and another ten scientists submitted a report on bubonic plague experiments using humans, along with thousands of the slides the Japanese had managed to spirit out of Manchuria before the Soviets had arrived. There were also 600 pages of secret articles written by Unit 731 scientists on human experimentation, germ warfare, and chemical warfare.[20]

Ishii and his confederates began to agitate for a more formal arrangement with the Americans, perhaps fearful that they would be handed over to the Soviets or placed on trial for war crimes once they had outlived their usefulness, and they asked for written guarantees they would be immune to prosecution forever, which was a step further from what MacArthur had offered them. 'If you will give me documentary immunity for myself, superiors, and subordinates, I can get all the information for you,' wrote Shiro Ishii confidently to the Americans. 'I would like to be hired by the US as a biological warfare expert. In the preparation for the war with Russia, I can give you the advantage of my 20 years research and experience.'[21] In this last statement he was not wide of the mark. Ishii's request was transmitted on 6 May 1947 to General MacArthur who passed it up the chain of command to the Pentagon. MacArthur, by now fully aware of the methods employed at Unit 731 in order to obtain the research material the Americans were so keen to lay their hands on, clearly had no qualms about the morality of the deal that he was negotiating, even commenting: 'Information about [human] vivisection useful.'[22] MacArthur also wrote to the War Department further outlining Ishii's potential usefulness: 'Ishii claims to have extreme theoretical high-level knowledge including strategic and tactical use of BW on defense and offense, backed by some research on best BW agents to employ by geographical areas of Far East, [and] the use of BW in cold climates.'[23]

As we have seen, at the time Ishii made his request for a written assurance, the Tokyo Trials were underway. Daniel Barenblatt, a leading authority on Unit 731, states that the authorities in Washington D.C. monitored the legal proceedings very carefully without committing to give Ishii an answer to his request for immunity at this stage. Evidently, the Americans wanted to see whether any biological warfare revelations would surface in open court after they had already ruled out their inclusion in the prosecution's case, meaning that they would swing with the prevailing wind and hand over Ishii and his confederates for trial if their Allies, including Britain, China and the Soviet Union, demanded it. In the meantime, the Pentagon sent more experts to Japan to carry out more interviews and to receive and catalogue a substantial haul of information from the cooperative Japanese.

Many former Unit 731 personnel remained cautious about coming forward and speaking to the Americans because they still believed that any information they provided would be passed on to their bitter enemy, the Soviets. The Japanese also claimed they were victims, and had been forced to develop biological weapons because they had discovered that the Soviets were conducting research into them. As we have seen, many senior Japanese officials denounced Ishii as a renegade who had operated outside of the legitimate military chain of command – a claim that was soon proven to be complete nonsense when it was discovered that Unit 731 was an integral and well-funded part of the Kwantung Army, deriving its authority from none other than Emperor Hirohito himself. There was also the blanket denial that members of the Japanese medical profession had helped Ishii, which was another lie, and that Emperor Hirohito had had absolutely no knowledge of the activities of Unit 731, another lie.

It has subsequently come to light that senior members of the Japanese Imperial Family visited Pingfan during the war and even witnessed human experiments first hand, and that films of those experiments had been personally delivered to the Imperial Palace in Tokyo by an employee of Unit 731. They were handed directly to representatives of the Imperial Household Agency, the government department that looks after the Imperial Family.

Regardless of all the lies, the Japanese soon realised that cooperation with the Americans was actually quite a good thing. The American attitude towards a defeated foe was very different from what they had been told to expect, and it encouraged their cooperation. 'During the war, Japanese civilians had been bombed, burned, and irradiated. American conduct from the beginning of the Occupation though, had consistently demonstrated that the Japanese now would be treated in an orderly and compassionate manner.'[24] Apart from the fear of being handed over to the Soviets, Ishii and his comrades also feared being sent back to China. MacArthur's pressure on the War Department to grant the Unit 731 scientists immunity ultimately succeeded, largely because it was such an easy decision to make. The Americans weighed the benefits of sending Ishii and his comrades to trial in Tokyo against the benefits of pardoning the senior Japanese researchers. The granting of immunity meant that the fascinating biological weapons data held by the Japanese would not come out in open court, enabling the Soviets and America's allies to obtain it. When the pardon was granted, Washington was no longer in the dark concerning Shiro Ishii's wartime activities. One of the reasons for this clarity was the Soviets who had actually handed over the transcripts of their interrogations of Unit 731 personnel in Khabarovsk to the Americans. MacArthur advised the War Department that these transcripts 'confirm authenticity of USSR interrogation and indicate Japanese activity in (a) Human experimentation. (b) Field trial against Chinese. (c) Large scale program. (d) Research on BW by crop destruction. (e) Possible that Japanese General Staff knew and authorized program. (f) Thought and research devoted to strategic and tactical use of BW ... Above topics are of great intelligence value to us.'[25]

On 3 June 1947 officials in Washington D.C. contacted Alva C. Carpenter of the SCAP Legal Section. They wanted to weigh the evidence against Ishii and his subordinates relating to war crimes. Washington wanted to know which of the Allied nations had filed war crimes charges against Ishii and the other Unit 731 veterans. Carpenter informed Washington that the only 'evidence' that he held consisted of anonymous letters, hearsay affidavits and rumours. In Carpenter's opinion, they 'do not reveal sufficient evidence to support war crimes charges. The alleged victims are of unknown identity. Unconfirmed allegations are to the effect that criminals, farmers, women and children were used for BW experimental purposes.'[26] Once again, the allegations that had been reported to SCAP by the Japanese Communist Party were repeated, which in part noted that Unit 731 'conducted experimentation on captured Americans in Mukden and that simultaneously, research on similar lines was conducted in Tokyo and Kyoto.'[27] Carpenter was not being entirely accurate in stating his opinion about the 'evidence' held by his office. On 17 April 1946 Osamu Hataba, a Japanese veteran of Unit 1644, a sub-division of Unit 731 based in Nanking, submitted a written affidavit to David Sutton, an IPS investigator in Shanghai. Hataba had been so disgusted and sickened by the activities of Unit 1644 he had defected to the Chinese Nationalist Army during the latter part of the war. His affidavit outlined Japanese attacks in 1943 on Chinese population centres using disease bombs and research into poisons. On 29 April 1946 another former Unit 1644 man, the equally guilt-stricken Hasane Hari, submitted another written affidavit that further outlined human experimentation and more details of the disease campaign unleashed against Chinese civilians.

Of course, had they wanted to, the Americans could have laid the above allegations alongside the transcripts of the interrogations of Major Tomio Karasawa, the Unit 731 section chief, that had been given to them by the Soviets. These contained direct allegations of experiments on American POWs. President Harry S. Truman was kept informed of these American investigations and moves around the Unit 731 personnel, and evidently backed General MacArthur's and the War Department's decision to grant Ishii and his comrades immunity from prosecution.

The affidavits submitted by Hataba and Hari were not used at the Tokyo trials and neither was the Soviet interrogation transcript of Major Karasawa. In fact, the activities of Unit 731 were only mentioned once during the course of the trials but created quite a stir in the court. However, the defence counsels' took advantage of the admission by claiming that such allegations were simply too inhumane to be true. The Chief Judge, Australian Sir William Webb, stated that such statements, as made by the prosecution, were 'mere assertion unsupported by any evidence'[28]. This attitude certainly assisted the defence and it was enough to quash the issue of Unit 731 permanently during the trials, and the Americans undoubtedly breathed a sigh of relief after that particular judicial hurdle had been deftly jumped. The Soviets were particularly annoyed by the American attitude, especially after they had furnished the State Department with the details of the interrogations of Unit 731 personnel. As Hal Gold writes: 'One might raise the question of what role the transfer of Japan's biological warfare potential to the US played in pushing the Soviets to outdo America in nuclear capability.'[29]

By 1947, the Americans had begun to cooperate a little more with the British concerning what they were learning about the Japanese biological warfare programme, including agreeing to an exchange of personnel between Camp Detrick and Porton Down, the secret British BW research facility. Major General Alden Waitt, who between 1945 and 1949 was Chief of the US Army Chemical Corps, the unit charged with disseminating the secrets of Unit 731 and creating America's own weapons of mass destruction, attended joint meetings with his British counterparts in the UK. Waitt admitted at one meeting 'that in the course of War Crimes Prosecution in the Far East most important evidence had come to light regarding experiments which had been carried out by the Japanese with B.W. agents.' In recapitulating the conclusions of a preliminary report, he expressed the view that 'a full study of the comprehensive evidence now available might lead to considerable revisions of current views on B.W.' In other words, the Americans were prepared to give the British a peek at the incredible deluge of BW research material that they had collected from Dr. Ishii and his associates, hinting that it would transform British understanding of biological warfare. The report ends with the understatement: 'THE MEETING took note with interest.'[30]

In September 1947, when the Americans informed Dr. Naito of General MacArthur's final decision to grant him and his friends immunity in writing in return for them 'spilling the beans' about Unit 731, Naito was naturally overjoyed. 'This made a deep impression, and the data came in waves after that,' recorded the American interrogators, '... we could hardly keep up with it.'[31] In order to secure Ishii, and to protect him, the American occupation authorities made a direct move. He was placed under house arrest and Lieutenant-Colonel Arvo Thompson personally grilled him on many occasions, trying to penetrate the labyrinthine organisational structure of Unit 731, unravel the weapons research from the civilian medical research that had been conducted and make sense of the mountain of data that he and his colleagues were receiving from the Japanese.

Although the Americans successfully kept revelations about Unit 731 out the courtroom in Tokyo, they did pursue the prosecution of the Kyushu University professors and their assistants who had performed grisly and terminal vivisection experiments on the eight members of the B-29 Superfortress that was shot down over Japan. Because the SCAP Legal Section in this case classified the defendants as 'Class B' or 'Class C' war criminals, little attention was paid to their trial in the Allied media, even when shocking and sickening revelations of cannibalism were also revealed during the course of the proceedings. On 27 August 1948 the US Military Court sentenced two of the Kyushu University professors to death for their part in the murders of the eight USAAF airmen. The rest of the defendants received prison terms that ranged from fifteen to twenty-five years. These sentences represented the Western Allies sole attempt to punish Japanese personnel associated with the activities of Unit 731. The only other trial of Unit 731 personnel was conducted deep behind the Iron Curtain in the Soviet Union in 1949.

The two Kyushu University doctors who were sentenced to hang never did so. One cheated death by the rope by committing suicide in prison, while the other had his sentence commuted to life imprisonment. He was released in the mid-1950s alongside all other Japanese war criminals. During the course of the trial, the mountain of deaths caused by similar experiments conducted by the Japanese in Manchuria was never mentioned even once, ensuring that no link was made between what had occurred at the Kyushu University campus in Fukuoka and at Pingfan, even though they were intimately and institutionally linked. The American cover-up was, by 1948, firmly in place.

Although basically a show trial, the Soviet Union should at least be commended for actually putting some of the Unit 731 criminals on trial. The trial at Khabarovsk was made possible because the USSR managed to lay their hands on twelve Japanese personnel who were intimately involved in the activities at Pingfan. They were swept up when the Red Army had overrun Manchuria in August 1945 and taken the surrender of the Kwantung Army. These dozen men were placed on trial in Siberia in 1949 as part of a propaganda ploy to embarrass the United States and to extract some measure of Cold War vengeance for denying the Soviets biological warfare secrets. When the Soviets realised the Americans had most of the Japanese biological warfare programme working for them, the furious Soviets decided to try and shame the Americans by having the few captured Unit 731 personnel in their hands spell out the heinous nature of their crimes to the world, testimony that included some of the first references to experiments on Allied POWs. A book of the trial transcript was even published in English in Moscow[32], but the whole show was dismissed as Communist propaganda in the West. The subsequent prison sentences that the Soviet court handed down to the Japanese in their custody were just, but extremely lenient, considering the crimes that they stood accused of:

1. General Otozo Yamada, former Commander-in-Chief, Kwantung Army – 25 years
2. Lieutenant General Ryuji Kajitsuka, former Chief of Medical Administration, Kwantung Army – 25 years
3. Lieutenant General Takaatsu Takahashi, former Chief of Veterinary Service, Kwantung Army – 25 years
4. Major Tomio Karasawa, former section chief, Unit 731 – 18 years
5. Lieutenant-Colonel Toshihide Nishi, former division chief, Unit 731 – 20 years
6. Major Masao Onoue, former branch chief, Unit 731 – 12 years
7. Major General Shuniji Sato, former Chief of Medical Service, 5th Army – 20 years
8. Lieutenant Zensaku Hirazakura, former researcher, Unit 100 – 10 years
9. Senior Sergeant Kazuo Mitomo, former member of Unit 100 – 15 years
10. Corporal Norimitsu Kikuchi, former medical orderly, Branch 643, Unit 731 – 2 years
11. Private Yuji Kurushima, former laboratory orderly, Branch 162, Unit 731 – 3 years

All of those found guilty at Khabarovsk were repatriated to Japan in 1956 and able to begin new lives as free men.

The Devil's Doctors

The American response to the Khabarovsk trial was predictable enough. It was denounced as 'communist propaganda' and the charges were dismissed as groundless and not based on any evidence other than hearsay. The fact that the Americans had been more than happy to receive copies of the NKVD interrogation transcripts from the Soviets when they had been trying to ascertain the importance of the documentary evidence they had been receiving from Naito and Ishii, was quietly ignored in the interests of national security. The public blanket denial of the existence of Unit 731, or of human experimentation, by the American government extended to rubbishing Major Kawasawa's assertion that American POWs at Mukden were used in human experiments. The entire testimony was dismissed as an NKVD fabrication.

Daniel Barenblatt notes that in 1982 the Soviet material was reassessed and seen for the first time as a painfully truthful and accurate picture of the different types of crimes committed at the various Unit 731 stations. The last surviving Allied judge from the Tokyo Trials, B.V.A. Roling of the Netherlands, expressed his surprise when he was told about Unit 731. He stated that the Tokyo judges had never heard of Dr. Ishii or of his nefarious unit during the course of the trials. Roling was particularly incensed by the American cover-up that had occurred in the 1940s. He said that the Americans ought to 'be ashamed because of the fact they withheld information from the Court with respect to the biological experiments of the Japanese in Manchuria on Chinese and American prisoners of war.'[33] But, by the time Roling spoke out it was all too little, too late, as far as examining seriously the claims of experiments on Allied POWs. The Japanese scientists involved had mostly risen to senior positions in postwar Japanese society and many, including Ishii, had actively worked on sensitive and top secret research for the United States. These men were, to all intents and purposes, virtual untouchables.

Ishii settled in Maryland where he worked on bio-weapons research for the American military until he died of throat cancer in 1959. Others slipped back into Japan once their work was completed in America. These included a prominent Unit 731 doctor, Masaji Kitano, who went on to be president of Japan's largest pharmaceutical company, Green Cross.[34] It would be the equivalent of the notorious Auschwitz war criminal Dr. Josef Mengele sitting on the board of directors of Bayer Healthcare or Glaxo Smith Kline. Other Japanese officers active in Unit 731 went on to fabulous postwar careers, including one who became the Governor of Tokyo, another who was President of the Japan Medical Association, and one who was head of the Japan Olympic Committee. So much for Ishii's admonition to them at the end of the war to stay out of the limelight.

Chapter 10

Operation 'PX'

> *While it is highly probable that local Japanese Commanders will continue to exercise discretion in using their reserves of CW [Chemical Warfare] ammunition or even in using any limited resources in BW [Biological Warfare] within their reach, it is NOT considered likely that either CW or BW will be inflicted by Japan on a strategic scale.*
>
> Professor G.D. Murray, War Cabinet
> Bacteriological Warfare Committee, 1944

A single engine Japanese Navy aircraft banked sharply in the skies over San Francisco, as inaccurate puffs of ack-ack fire blossomed in the clear blue sky. Following closely behind the first plane were two others, and the three of them banked noisily over the downtown of the American metropolis after releasing their bombs. On the ground there had not been any explosions, even though people had seen dark cylindrical shapes detach themselves from the aircraft and tumble between the tall buildings. The only noise was the high-pitched shriek of aero engines and the steady thumping of anti-aircraft guns in the Bay Area. At ground level, air raid wardens and firefighters spotted one of the 'bombs' lying in a street not far from an abandoned tram. It had shattered like a grey painted egg. Strange pellets had been widely dispersed on the ground, but other than that everything appeared normal. The emergency workers considered it a dud, and although the Japanese attack was sudden and audacious, no damage had been caused. What they did not know was that the air, so clear and warm, was alive with an invisible killer, and with every breath the citizens of the city took, they risked drawing a terrible disease deep into their bodies. Within days thousands would sicken and begin to die, hospitals would overflow with casualties, and the city would cease to function as many thousands more tried to flee, clogging roads vital for the American war effort with sickened people. At every town and village refugees visited, more would become infected and die. Doomsday had come. Thankfully for everyone concerned, the preceding description were fictional – but what many people do not realise is how close fiction came to becoming a grim reality.

Shiro Ishii's 'weapons of mass destruction', devised, researched, and constructed at the cost of hundreds of thousands of lives, were never used against the Western Allies. But they did come very close to being deployed outside of China, and if they had been, the whole history of the war would probably have been quite different. It is perhaps worth examining how the Japanese military developed weapons that could deliver biological warfare devices directly on to the American mainland, as the war turned further and further against the nation. The Japanese seriously considered using them for a while, but in the end they realised that unleashing such terrible weapons against defenceless Chinese civilians was very different from unleashing them against a world power with virtually unlimited military potential and the ability to strike back directly at the Japanese mainland. In the end, the only thing that really prevented the deployment of Unit 731's biological weapons was the very real fear that the Americans might in return bomb Japan with their own ballistic germs. Little did the Japanese realise that the Americans had an even more serious weapon that they were preparing to use on the Japanese civilian population – the atomic bomb.

The development and deployment of biological warfare delivery platforms by the Japanese is one of those fascinating 'what if' scenarios of the Second World War. They demonstrate there was a clear link between Unit 731 and the science of warfare, and that the Japanese recognised the types of biological weapons developed and tested by Shiro Ishii in Manchuria could represent a last ditch effort to stave off a humiliating and total defeat. In attempting to prevent this inevitable surrender, Japanese scientists and military officers were quite inventive in their determination to take the fight to the enemy's home turf. For a nation with only one tenth of the industrial capacity of its main enemy (and by the latter part of the war this had already been severely eroded by the American strategic bombing campaign against industrial centres, as well as the Allied submarine campaign against Japan's merchant marine), it represented an extremely ambitious plan, and, incredibly, it very nearly succeeded.

In 1942, a submarine-launched Japanese spotter plane that flew not much faster than a speeding car, dropped some small incendiary bombs over the forests of Oregon in the United States. The Japanese plan had been to create massive forest fires in the Pacific Northwest which would have caused huge material damage, destroyed countless communities, and have struck a blow against American morale. The plan failed, largely because the forests had been recently drenched by rain. The Japanese tried again a few days later, with the same result.[1]

The Japanese High Command acknowledged that although the overall objectives of the fire-bombing operation were sound, the two sorties that had been made over Oregon by navy pilot Chief Warrant Officer Nobuo Fujita had led to negligible results. A massive effort was required to transport one very small aircraft across the Pacific on board an extremely valuable submarine, to drop a tiny amount of bombs. At best it would have proved an amazing propaganda coup had the United States authorities realized that Japan had successfully attacked the American mainland, but very little media coverage emerged. Another munitions delivery system was required, and this time Japanese scientists decided upon an unmanned and very economical option – the paper balloon.

The Japanese initially required utilization of their submarine force once again to attack the United States, and in 1943 some two hundred balloons were carefully prepared. The balloons were to be launched towards the American mainland from two modified submarines, the *I-34* and *I-35*. Each balloon had a twenty-foot envelope, and a range of more than six hundred miles. Although the operation was fully prepared by August 1943, the Imperial Japanese Navy soon realised that employing submarines on such missions would not have been a sensible use of their potential, especially as the war had long since begun to go against Japan. The project was shelved, and the navy dropped balloon bomb

Operation 'PX'

research altogether. The Imperial Japanese Army, however, continued development in secret. As the army had no submarines which could be used to launch balloons from a mid-point in the Pacific between Japan and the United States, the new weapons had to be designed to depart from the Japanese homeland itself.

The army balloon-bomb project, codenamed Operation *'Fugo'* (Windship Weapon), was based at the 9th Military Technical Research Institute under the command of Major General Sueyoshi Kusaba. The researchers worked in cooperation with scientists from the Central Meteorological Observatory in Tokyo and produced a balloon design they designated the Type-A. It was ingeniously constructed from sixty-four laminated mulberry tree paper gores (the sections forming the curved surface of the balloon). This was glued together with a form of potato paste to form a balloon envelope with a 100-foot circumference. The envelope was filled with 19,000 cubic feet of hydrogen to provide the balloon with the necessary high ceiling to carry it across the Pacific to America. Below the envelope was suspended a woven Dural ring with bombs and thirty-six ballast sandbags attached, controlled by three aneroid barometers and a C (small) battery mounted on a platform above the ring that controlled a circuit to maintain altitude, and to release the bombs. Each balloon carried a payload of two 11-pound thermalite incendiary bombs and one 33-pound anti-personnel fragmentation bomb. At this point, the Japanese were not proposing fitting the balloons with Shiro Ishii's ceramic 'germ bombs', but the process would not have presented undue difficulties. Of course, any switch to germ bombs would have necessitated a change in targets, as it would have been desirable for the balloons to release their payloads over high-density population centres, such as Los Angeles and San Francisco. Naturally, hitting vast forests with largely uncontrollable balloons was going to be a lot easier. The Japanese called the resulting new weapon *fusen bakudan* or 'fire bombs'. Launch sites were located on the east coast of the Japanese island of Honshu, at Otsu, Ichinomiryu and Nakaso.

Once released, the balloons travelled at the behest of the wind, and carried to the North American continent on high altitude currents, cruising in the Jet Stream at between 20,000 and 40,000 feet. To maintain this very high altitude during flight, sand was automatically released from the ballast bags if the balloon began to sink lower. In the daytime the balloon would cruise at its maximum altitude, but at night the balloon envelope would collect dew and slowly sink as it became progressively heavier. When this happened, the on-board altimeter would cause a set of blow plugs to fire, releasing some of the sandbag ballast and thereby restoring the balloon's altitude. It was another simple, yet highly effective, device. When all of the sand was dumped the bombs themselves would become the final ballast, and they were released automatically – an event calculated to occur over the mainland of the United States. Finally, a picric acid block would explode, destroying the balloon gondola; with a fuse being lit that was connected to a charge on the balloon itself. The resultant mixture of hydrogen, air and explosives would cause the balloon envelope to burn up as a large orange fireball, destroying any evidence of its manufacture, origin and payload delivery method. Because the balloons cruised at such a high altitude, observers on the ground could not see them with ease, and most American interceptor aircraft of the period found it difficult to climb to the highest balloon cruising altitudes to shoot them down. All in all, it was a simple, cheap, but extremely ingenious weapon, that had the potential to rain death and destruction onto the American mainland, and a weapon that was to make the American authorities extremely nervous.

The first balloon launch occurred on 3 November 1944. Two days later a US Navy patrol boat discovered a mysterious balloon floating in the sea sixty-six miles off San Pedro, California. The first recorded successful attack on the United States occurred on 6 December 1944, when bombs were dropped around twelve miles southwest of Owl Creek Mountain, close to Thermopolis in Wyoming. Fragments of balloon envelopes and gondolas were discovered in Alaska and Montana, and forensic tests soon confirmed that the wreckage was of Japanese origin.[2] The question for the authorities was how the Japanese were delivering these weapons to the United States? The American people were not informed of the attacks, and the media was ordered not to report this sinister new development for fear of spreading panic.

The United States quickly developed counter-measures to deal with this unique threat, codenamed 'Operation Firefly.' The US 4th Air Force gathered fighter squadrons equipped with aircraft capable of reaching very high altitudes that were sent aloft to

Operation 'PX'

shoot down the balloons before they could release their payloads, and many were downed over the Aleutian Islands as they sank to lower altitudes in their journey east. One was shot down over Oregon. Interestingly, it appears to have been the Americans who first thought the Japanese could use the balloons to deliver chemical and biological warfare agents to the United States, and to counter any such threat stocks of decontamination chemicals were quietly distributed to the Western states, and farmers were asked to report any strange crop markings or animal infections that occurred. The American authorities deliberately played down the potential damage that the balloon bombs could have wreaked, Lyle Watts of the Agricultural Department commenting in June 1945 that the forest service was 'less worried about this Japanese balloon attack than we are with matches and smokes in the hands of good Americans hiking and camping in the woods.'[3] Further precautions were taken and a US Army unit, the 555th Parachute Infantry Battalion (nicknamed the 'Triple Nickle' because of their unit number), was trained to act as fire jumpers should the incendiary bombs set the forests ablaze.

Of the 9,300 balloons launched from Japan, only 212 were confirmed as having actually arrived in the United States and Mexico, landing as far east as Michigan, and a further seventy-three were confirmed to have come down in Canada. The only fatalities caused by the balloon bombs occurred on 5 May 1945, on Gearhart Mountain, near Bly, Oregon, when a picnicking party of one adult and five children was tragically killed after dragging an unexploded Japanese 15-kg anti-personnel bomb out of the woods. These six people are the only known fatalities caused by enemy action on the mainland of the United States during the Second World War.[4] It is not known whether any of the balloon bombs started forest fires, as was intended.

In April 1945 the Japanese ceased their balloon launches, largely because they believed that the campaign was a complete failure owing to a lack of balloon-bomb-related news stories in the American media. What remains certain, however, is the fact that many of the bombs remain unaccounted for and today remain scattered over the American countryside, as-yet undiscovered and potentially lethal relics of a conflict that ended over six decades ago.

While the balloon-bombing campaign was a failure, the Japanese were not yet prepared to admit defeat when it came to launching attacks on the United States. What was required was a much more-potent weapons delivery system that could be directed accurately against specific targets, rather than leaving the results to luck. Even before the balloon-bomb campaign was terminated, the Imperial Japanese Navy was working in secret to make that new weapons system a reality – and this time the deployment of biological weapons was discussed at the very highest levels of the Japanese high command, and a nefarious and deadly plan was created to reign down death and destruction on the American people.

'Japan, while morally more likely to employ the BW [Biological Warfare] weapon, is physically far less capable of wielding it effectively [compared with Nazi Germany],'[5] wrote Professor G.D. Murray, a top British biological warfare scientist to the War Cabinet on 31 July 1944. Murray could not conceive of Japan possessing the technology or the wherewithal to launch a biological warfare attack on the Allies. 'No vital and primary Allied centre of industry and activity is within range of her fleet or bomber craft. In any case, these two arms of Japan have lost nearly every vestige of tactical and strategic supremacy even in their home waters.'[6] What Professor Murray ignored was the one area where Japan still possessed some advantages – the design and production of long-range submarines. Even as Winston Churchill and the War Cabinet in Whitehall were reading Professor Murray's report, the Japanese were busy bringing into existence the ideal platform upon which they could reign down biological holocaust upon the United States, if they had so chosen. In fact, they held in their hands the ability to transform the whole course of the war, and certainly to have brought real suffering to the American home front. What Professor Murray also did not know was the willingness of the Japanese military to use biological weapons in a last ditch attempt to stave off an inevitable defeat.

In a brilliant operation that involved Shiro Ishii at the highest levels of planning, the Japanese were determined to combine all of the elements of their previous germ bomb attacks on Chinese towns and cities with an ingenious new delivery system. If carried out, the Japanese plan would have gone down in history as one of the worst war crimes ever committed.

In 1944, the Allies did not know very much about Shiro Ishii's vast complex at Pingfan, nor how advanced Japan had become in

OPERATION 'PX'

producing viable biological weapons. It was all deeply mysterious, though unsettling. The temptation among Allied analysts was to portray Japan as an inferior foe as compared with Nazi Germany, and this assessment would later be proved quite wrong. 'Her scientific and industrial resources are minimal in comparison with Germany or with the three leading United Nations,' wrote Professor Murray. 'While it is highly probable that local Japanese Commanders will continue to exercise discretion in using their reserves of CW [Chemical Warfare] ammunition or even in using any limited resources in BW within their reach, it is NOT considered likely that either CW or BW will be inflicted by Japan on a strategic scale.'[7]

The Japanese realised that if they really wanted to take the fight to the American mainland, which hitherto had been protected from the effects of the war by its distance from the two Axis powers, they would have to devise some new and unique machine to make this possible. Japan's submarine construction programme eventually was to produce the single most extraordinary class of boats conceived by any of the combatant navies of the Second World War. The *I-400* class submarines were created in order to take the Japanese plan to attack the United States on home ground to its devastating conclusion. As early as April 1942, the Imperial Japanese Navy had decided to order the construction of a class of submarine that would completely dwarf previous Japanese creations in order to provide a far-reaching strike capacity. What was needed was a single submarine that was both large enough to reach land targets in the United States without requiring any refuelling, and was able to carry more than one aircraft with which to launch attacks when it got there. The new bombers would have to be potent weapons as well, able to deliver a large payload of bombs, but still retaining floatplane characteristics that would enable their operation at sea by a surfaced submarine. In effect, the Japanese navy required a submarine aircraft carrier, and this is exactly what they set about designing and constructing between April 1942 and December 1944.

Each *I-400* class vessel was a monster; the largest submarines built until well into the Cold War, and their size only surpassed in 1962 when the Americans commissioned the USS *Lafayette*. Displacing 5,223-tons surfaced, each boat was 400.3 feet in length. With a beam of 39.3 feet, each vessel was powered by four diesel engines and electric motors. Atop the weather deck was a 115-foot long waterproof hanger twelve feet wide and capacious enough for *three* specially designed torpedo-bombers. In front of the hangar, bolted to the immense deck, stretched a pneumatic aircraft-launching catapult eighty-five feet in length, and alongside this a powerful hydraulic crane for recovering the aircraft from the sea.[8] The Imperial Navy had copied the snorkel technology that was fitted to late-war German U-boats, and these were fitted to all four of the *I-400* class submarines. The snorkel mast, when extended above the surface of the water as the submarine cruised at periscope depth, enabled the boat to run on diesel engines instead of batteries, producing a greatly increased underwater speed and protection from aerial detection and attack.

The *I-400* class submarines were quite fast, capable of a top surface or submerged snorkel speed of 18.7 knots, or if fully submerged and running on their electric motors, 6.5 knots. Radar and radar detectors, though not of a superior German standard, were fitted to all four boats of the class. Although primarily launch platforms for aircraft, each boat was more than capable of fighting like any other submarines, having eight torpedo tubes and an improved 140mm 50-calibre deck gun. Improved anti-aircraft defences increased each boat's chances of standing off an aerial assault, with a 25mm cannon mounted on the conning tower, and three triple barrel 25mm cannons located on top of the aircraft hangar. With a maximum diving depth of almost 330 feet, each boat took slightly under one minute to perform an emergency crash-dive.[9] Hugely capacious fuel tanks on each of the boats meant that these submarine aircraft carriers were capable of cruising an astounding *35,500* nautical miles at 14 knots before the tanks ran dry; in other terms giving the Japanese skipper the ability to circumnavigate the globe one-and-a-half times. The huge range of these vessels meant that for the first time in the war the Japanese Navy had a machine capable of not only crossing the Pacific to attack the West Coast of the United States, but also, in theory, of crossing into the Atlantic Ocean via Cape Horn and unleashing air strikes against New York or Washington D.C. Both cities were later considered by naval planners in Tokyo for attacks. If the strike aircraft were fitted with Shiro Ishii's specially designed ceramic germ bombs, the devastation that could have been wrought against the urban populations of America's most

OPERATION 'PX'

important cities does not bare thinking about. The concomitant damage that could have been done to American war production if, for example, bubonic plague had been released all over the largest production centres on the East and West coasts, could have been significant, and perhaps enough to have altered the course of the war in Japan's favour.

Such superb and powerful vessels required an equally superb and capable aircraft type to operate from them, and here the Japanese also excelled. Each submarine was designed to carry a maximum of three Aichi M6A1 *Seiran* torpedo bombers. *Seiran* can be roughly translated from the Japanese as 'Storm from the sky', and these aircraft were extremely sturdy birds of destruction. Although still configured as floatplanes, each monoplane measured thirty-five feet in length, with a wingspan of forty feet. Designed by Toshio Ozaki, chief engineer at Aichi, the *Seiran* had to conform to a series of strict guidelines laid down by the Imperial Navy as they sought the perfect plane for their new submarines. In late 1942 Ozaki began developing the aircraft the navy specified must have been capable of carrying a maximum bomb load consisting of a single 1,288-lb (800kg) aerial bomb or torpedo. If a *kamikaze* mission was called for, because of Japan's deteriorating strategic position, the aircraft floats could be detached and the fuel and bomb load increased for a one-way mission against the enemy. Under normal, non-*kamikaze*, operating conditions each *Seiran* had a range of 654 miles, which meant that the 'mother' submarine could stand some way off from the enemy shore when launching and recovering it's air group, instead of having to come close inshore to launch and then sit vulnerably on the surface awaiting an aircraft's return from its sortie. When at sea, the *Seiran* aircraft were stored inside the huge deck hangar with their floats detached and their wings and tails folded up. All three bombers could be assembled, fuelled, and fitted with either torpedoes or aerial bombs (including germ bombs), attached to the launching ramp and sent aloft in only forty-five minutes.

The first prototype *Seiran* was completed in October 1943 and several others followed. In early 1944, full production was ordered before final testing had been completed at Aichi. This decision was forced upon the Japanese by the deteriorating naval situation and the necessity of getting the new submarines and aircraft into action as soon as possible. This was to prove to be no easy task as

American bombing raids and even an earthquake conspired to completely shut down production at Aichi by March 1945. Aichi engineers were only able to cobble together twenty-six *Seiran* torpedo-bombers (including the prototypes) and a pair of land-based trainers. The navy no longer required a large number of *Seiran* aircraft as they had been forced by the weakening of Japan's economy to also scale back the number of *I-400* class submarines. The *I-400* was commissioned on 30 December 1944 and the *I-401* followed a few days later. The duties of the *I-402* were changed and she was refitted as a submarine fuel tanker. Two other boats, *I-404* and *I-405*, were abandoned on the slips and they were not completed before the Japanese surrender in August 1945.

The *I-400* and *I-401* were transferred into a new unit alongside two modified AM class submarines, the *I-13* and *I-14*. Originally this type of boat had only been capable of carrying a single float-plane but while they were under construction in 1944 the Japanese changed their plans and altered the configuration of the boats to accommodate two *Seiran* bombers. Under the overall command of Captain Tatsunosuke Ariizumi, the submarines were organized as 1st Submarine Flotilla, with the aircraft and aircrew forming 631st Air Corps. The *I-13* and *I-14* would each carry two aircraft, while the two *I-400*-class boats were loaded with full air groups of three *Seiran* bombers each. If launched in concert, the Japanese Navy could have put ten bombers over any city of its choosing, or have launched simultaneous strikes against several coastal cities without any warning.

It was at this point, with their new submarines ready for action, that elements in the Japanese High Command advocated using the aircraft to drop bubonic plague, cholera, dengue fever, typhus or a wide variety of other equally virulent germs on the United States in order to create widespread infection and panic. It was realised that the impact of only a small number of such bombs would have been devastating in comparison with the puny conventional bomb loads that the aircraft could carry. The leading advocate of the germ warfare plan was Vice-Admiral Jisaburo Ozawa, who was then the Vice Chief of the Naval General Staff in Tokyo. Along with his subordinates Ozawa formulated a plan that was codenamed 'Operation PX'.

One of the senior naval officers involved in formulating Operation 'PX', Captain Yoshio Eno, spoke out about the plan for the first time in 1977, saying that '... at the time, Japan was losing badly, and any means to win would have been all right.'[10] From the beginning, Operation 'PX' was conceived as a joint Army-Navy project. The senior Imperial Army representative was Colonel Takushiro Hattori. When the plan was first proposed before the Naval General Staff in Tokyo at the end of December 1944, two main drawbacks were immediately highlighted. Firstly, the Navy lacked data regarding the intended pathogens that would be used, and, secondly, they lacked the actual pathogens. Lieutenant-General Ishii was brought in to solve these two problems, which he swiftly did, recognising that the research that had been undertaken at Pingfan would find its practical expression in the annihilation of the hated Americans where they felt safest – in America itself. It was the chance of a lifetime for the ambitious Ishii. It would also vindicate all of the extensive research Ishii and Unit 731 had undertaken over nearly two decades into weaponising deadly pathogenic bacteria. In many aspects, Operation 'PX' could have been Unit 731's finest hour as far as Ishii and his colleagues were concerned. The plan was finalised on 26 March 1945, and appeared to be unstoppable. We can be sure the data that Unit 731 researchers had carefully collected concerning the immunity of Caucasians to various pathogens was now to come in to its own, including perhaps data gleaned from the POWs at Mukden Camp.

The Japanese military during the Second World War has often been portrayed as being led by rabid fanatics who cared little for the consequences of their actions, and instead were prepared to pursue ultimate victory at absolutely any cost in lives and material. To some extent, this is an accurate portrait, but even within a military as morally bankrupt as the Imperial Army and Navy, some voices of caution did still remain in the waning days of the war, and they now spoke out strongly against initiating Operation 'PX'. A leading and very influential member of the opposition to 'PX' was the army's most senior officer, General Yoshijiro Umezu. In his role as Chief of the General Staff, Umezu managed to deftly quash the plan on the very day it was finished, 26 March 1945, and certainly before any move was made to carry it out. It was a major blow for Ishii, Ozawa and cohorts. Umezu later explained why he felt compelled to terminate 'PX', an operation which if successful would have struck a very heavy blow indeed against the United States. 'If bacteriological warfare is conducted, it will grow from the dimension of war between Japan and America to an endless battle of humanity against bacteria. Japan will earn the derision of the world.'[11] Although General Ishii, Colonel Hattori, Captain Eno and the other officers who had been responsible for conceiving and planning Operation 'PX' vociferously objected to Umezu's decision, there was nothing they could do and the project was permanently shelved. Umezu clearly had seen the way the wind was blowing for Japan.

Although 'PX' was dropped, the Imperial Navy still wanted to launch its ten *Seiran* aircraft against targets in America, but this time armed with conventional weapons. Various targets were placed before the naval staff, including San Francisco, New York and Washington D.C., as well as the vital Panama Canal. The Navy eventually decided that a strike against the Panama Canal would have had the greatest effect on America's ability to prosecute the war against Japan, but in the end even this proposed operation, for which extensive training had begun, was scrapped and the Japanese High Command decided instead to expend the submarines and aircraft on useless *kamikaze* attacks on the US Navy's anchorage at Ulithi Atoll. Fortunately for everyone concerned, Japan surrendered before the aircraft could be launched.

We can only surmise that perhaps some of the data which emerged from Japanese experiments on Allied POWs and Russian civilians was useful during the planning of Operation 'PX'. It would certainly appear sensible and logical to suggest that it was, and it would fit in with Unit 731 research intent on discovering whether Caucasian prisoners suffered the same symptoms as Asian test subjects when exposed to various diseases. We can probably be sure that the Japanese who planned the operation knew which pathogens would have been most effective against a white population after conducting so many experiments on Caucasian prisoners both at Pingfan, and at other sites, including, perhaps, the Mukden Prisoner of War Camp. We cannot know for certain how much of the data that was derived from Unit 731's experiments on Allied personnel influenced the decision to launch a biological warfare attack on the United States, but we can be sure Shiro Ishii most definitely knew what the results would have been. Although General Umezu took the secret of Operation 'PX' with him to his grave, he saved a huge number of American lives

Operation 'PX'

by taking a firm stand against such a mad plan. The only caveat to this statement may be whether Umezu would have stopped 'PX' had he had advance warning of the American use of the atomic bomb against Japan.

Chapter 11

Dark Harvest

My husband set off for work at Porton Down on September 20, 1966. When I saw him that night he was in a terrible state; he had agonising stomach pains. He said, 'I've had that bloody American bubonic plague injection.' Three months later he died. I was told he had died of stomach cancer but I know they gave him a cocktail of 19 injections of smallpox, anthrax, plague, and polio over five years. I was told that he needed the immunisation jabs but I believe that was just an excuse. They were using him as a guinea pig. He wouldn't have refused because he would have been afraid to lose his job.[1]

Hettie Nyman

Unit 731 has cast a very long shadow over modern China. Its memory is constantly recycled and referred to during the endless diplomatic spats between the nation and its old enemy, Japan. It is not only words which still have the power to harm. The detritus of Shiro Ishii's mad experiments are still injuring people, even in the early twenty-first century. For example, in August 2003 twenty-nine local people living in Heilongjiang Province (formerly a part of Manchuria) were taken to hospital after construction crews uncovered a stash of Japanese artillery shells loaded with chemicals from the Unit 731 factory. The Japanese had buried them at the war's end in an attempt to cover their trail. This incident opened up another row between China and Japan over Japan's wartime record, an issue that simmers away just below the surface between the two powerful neighbours and often threatens to erupt into protest and violence at any time.

The curator at the Unit 731 museum in Pingfan summed up the significance of both the facility and the atrocities carried out by the Japanese in its buildings when he said: 'This is not just a Chinese concern; it is a concern of humanity.' The vibrations of history continue to ring down the decades, and like ripples in a stagnant and poisoned pond, Unit 731 remains at the epicentre of a deep and dark secret that the Allied Powers tried to bury in 1945, and is one they have continued to protect up to the present day. Although Unit 731 and the heinous activities conducted there are quite well understood today, many important questions remain unanswered. The question of whether or not British soldiers were fed into the horrors of Unit 731 is unsettled, and unsettling and it has led successive British governments to simply ignore the evidence and issue blanket denials of any Japanese wrongdoing concerning our men who were held at the Mukden Camp. The government has also continued to embargo many important documents relating to biological warfare research that they conducted just after the war.

The British, like their American allies, eventually benefitted enormously from a massive biological and chemical warfare data windfall that came initially from the defeated Germans in 1945. Establishing whether the British also benefitted from Japanese human experimentation data is a lot harder to prove. My trawl through the files at The National Archives revealed that most of the relevant documents are still either classified almost *seven decades* after the end of the war, or incomplete, with pages that presumably contain sensitive material having been replaced with a card that states simply that the page has been retained by the Government. However, some clues as to the dissemination of Unit 731 data do remain in the files, leading to the suggestion that Shiro Ishii's experimentation results did find their way into research in Britain which was aimed at protecting the nation from a Soviet attack during the Cold War, and indeed, that such information continues to exercise a role in modern biological weapons research.

The British first experimented with chemical weapons in 1916 at the height of the First World War when the 'Royal Engineers

Experimental Station' was established at Porton Down on land slightly northeast of the small village of Porton, near Salisbury in Wiltshire. Porton Down has remained the nerve centre of British chemical and biological warfare research ever since. Today it houses the Defence Science and Technology Laboratory, an Executive Agency of the Ministry of Defence (MoD), and an above top-secret institution spread over a very carefully monitored 7,000 acres of English countryside. Within Porton Down is also located the Health Protection Agency's Centre for Emergency Preparedness and Response, as well as a small science park. To the northwest is the MoD Boscombe Down test range facility.

During the First World War the scientists at Porton Down created chlorine, phosgene and mustard gas for offensive use. During the Second World War there was considerable research into chemical weapons, for example nitrogen mustard, as well as biological weapons, including anthrax and botulinum toxin. In 1942 very successful anthrax tests were carried out using bio-weapons at Gruinard Island in Scotland. The British were concerned about the possible effects of anthrax on population centres, should the Germans have decided to use such weapons. Eighty sheep were taken to the seventy-six square-mile uninhabited island and exposed to a particularly virulent strain of anthrax developed at Oxford University. All of the animals soon died. Gruinard Island was so badly polluted by anthrax that it was placed under an indefinite quarantine and only declared safe in 1990 after the government had mounted an extensive cleanup operation which included the removal of the topsoil from the island.

After the war ended, the scientists at Porton Down conducted research into recently discovered Nazi nerve agents which included Tabun, Sarin and Soman. By 1952 the British made a major breakthrough when they developed VX Gas, an extremely lethal nerve agent. Considerable work was undertaken on defensive measures, including the rapid detection and decontamination of chemical and biological warfare agents. Voluntary human tests were conducted and there have been persistent allegations of unethical human experiments at Porton Down. The issue of exactly how voluntary the tests were has been raised by the support groups who have campaigned for greater transparency and proper answers after the deaths of loved ones at the facility.

Dark Harvest

The most prominent case to have come to public attention was the death of twenty-year-old RAF Leading Aircraftman Ronald Maddison in 1953, after he was exposed to the Sarin nerve agent as part of a toxicity test. Maddison, from County Durham, was one of around 3,400 postwar volunteers who submitted themselves to chemical weapons tests at Porton Down. It remains a very controversial episode in the history of British weapons research with many of the men who took part later claiming that they were tricked into it by the military and have suffered long-term health issues as a result of the experiments; a situation that is not dissimilar to the claims made by some of the American survivors of the Mukden Camp. The test that killed Maddison on 6 May 1953 involved him and four other volunteers sitting inside a gas chamber wearing respirators. Each man had a cloth draped over one of his arms which had been impregnated with 200mg of Sarin.

Sarin gas is described as an organophosphorus compound, a colourless, odourless liquid that has been classified as a 'weapon of mass destruction' by the United Nations. Since 1993 the Chemical Weapons Convention has outlawed the production and stockpiling of Sarin. Discovered by accident in Germany in 1938 by scientists who were trying to create stronger pesticides, Sarin has twice come to the attention of the media when it has been used as a weapon. In March 1988 Saddam Hussein unleashed a two-day Sarin attack on the Kurdish city of Halabja in northern Iraq, killing around five thousand of the city's 70,000 inhabitants. And in 1995 a religious sect in Japan released an impure form of Sarin on the Tokyo underground railway system, killing thirteen people and injuring dozens more.

Within twenty minutes of beginning the test Ronald Maddison had been told was to 'cure the common cold', he complained of feeling unwell. He then collapsed to the floor and began to convulse. Scientists immediately removed him from the chamber, took off his respirator, and injected him with atropine before he was rushed by ambulance to a nearby medical facility where he died. The Sarin had blocked the flow of air into Maddison's lungs, starving his brain and body of oxygen. An inquiry was immediately launched, but it was held in secret. On 16 May 1953 the death of Maddison was declared to have been 'misadventure'.

It was reported that the Ministry of Defence secretly paid Maddison's funeral expenses. However, that was not the end of the story. In July 1999 Wiltshire Constabulary – the police force that covers the area where Porton Down is located – launched Operation 'Antler' in an attempt to investigate the extent of malfeasance that had been committed at Porton Down over the decades since the Second World War. Altogether, the police found that Porton Down had employed around twenty thousand men as human guinea pigs before, during, and after the Second World War. The police interviewed 700 surviving veterans, many of whom claimed to have been tricked into signing up for the Service Volunteer Programme. When Maddison died in 1953, the MoD paid each volunteer 15 shillings – the equivalent of about £12.00 today – and threw in a three-day pass. It was a measly sum of money for the risks to life and limb that were involved. By 2004 Wiltshire Constabulary had drawn up twenty-five cases for possible prosecution and eventually forwarded eight to the Crown Prosecution Service. Unfortunately, the CPS decided that none of the scientists involved in the experiments at Porton Down would be prosecuted, and the cases were closed. The MoD agreed to pay the Maddison family £100,000 compensation in 2006 after a fresh inquest into the young airman's death returned a verdict of 'unlawful acts' in 2004.[2]

Research into chemical and biological warfare in Britain continues to the present day but it remains highly secret. Even Members of Parliament have been denied information about what goes on at Porton Down. One Conservative Member of Parliament, Colonel Patrick Mercer, recalled his own experience of the place when he was a young army officer. 'It was hideous, a hutted camp, where it seemed to do nothing but rain. There were a series of bunkers to which you were thrust from time to time to be gassed with CS gas and to go through ghastly exercises underground wearing a gas mask.'[3] Many veterans have spoken of strange experiments that they were a part of. 'As far as we were all concerned the tests were part of a programme searching for a cure for the common cold,' recalled former Fleet Air Arm storeman Eric Hatherall. It would be surprising to find a military establishment spending its budget on such a research project with no military potential. 'If I had though it was anything more than that I would not have put my name forward,' said Hatherall. 'They gave us each a glass of water and we were told to drink it, which I did, and I felt no adverse symptoms. It tasted like water to me, but some of the others who had taken the drink literally started trying to climb up the wall and cowering in corners. They were screaming and hallucinating and saying there were giant spiders in the room. It is now pretty obvious that they had been given LSD or another drug.'[4]

One thing known for certain is the very large scale of animal testing conducted at Porton Down. For example, the MoD reported in 2009 there were 8,168 'procedures' conducted against animals at the facility.[5] Pigs are routinely used for blast tests of explosives and other weapons to help develop personal protection equipment for front-line troops. Mice are used in the development of vaccines for microbial and viral infections, and various types of monkeys have been exposed to anthrax. This is only a sample of the types of experiments that are conducted at Porton Down, and of the species of animals used.

It has often been assumed the British automatically benefitted from information the Americans laid their hands on during the Second World War and during the later Cold War. Although they were the strongest of allies, and have remained so, the United States maintained a military lead over the rest of the world, partly by jealously guarding its secret technologies and the sources of this classified information. As we have already seen regarding General Douglas MacArthur's backstairs deal with Shiro Ishii and the Unit 731 scientists in Tokyo in 1946–47, the United States expressly forbade any dissemination of Japanese biological warfare data to the Soviet Union and was slow to give details to the British until it had had time to digest and make sense of the information. However, the British were certainly aware that the Japanese had been conducting extremely interesting research during the war, and that American agencies had managed to lay their hands upon it. The Americans, in fact, drip-fed the British with intriguing information that whetted Whitehall appetites for more.

I think it would be naïve to believe the British did not benefit from the information the Americans gained from the Japanese. The archives clearly show the Americans did pass documents to London, and that they also arranged exchanges of personnel between Camp Detrick and Porton Down. Whether any of the information passed from the Japanese to the Americans, and thence to the British, contained data that had been derived from experiments on American, British and Australian POWs at Mukden cannot be established at this time. And, it is fair to say that even if it was the case, we will never know the truth.

Conclusion

Autopsies being performed on the corpses by the visiting Japanese.

Major Robert Peaty, 15 February 1943

When all of the testimonies, documents and evidence presented throughout the course of this book are put together, it becomes difficult to deny that the treatment the Allied POWs received in the Mukden Camp in 1942–43 was a little strange, to say the least. On balance the *prima facie* evidence points to the Japanese having conducted medical tests on the prisoners at this camp. The witnesses, who reported extremely similar things at different times, and who were from several different nationalities, have inadvertently provided strong corroboration for each other's assertions. Perhaps it was all just coincidence? Perhaps what the prisoners witnessed was quite ordinary and was simply misinterpreted at the time, as most of them were not trained medical professionals and have commented with the benefit of hindsight. It may be easy to explain away the testimonies and memories of former prisoners-of-war on an individual basis, but it becomes more difficult to deny the admission of experiments made quite openly by several Japanese veterans of Unit 731. Why would they have lied? It served absolutely no purpose to do so, and indeed they ran the risk of punishment for their admissions.

If we believe the American and British governments' official views on this matter, we have to accept that the prisoners held at the Mukden Camp were treated no better or worse than any other Allied POWs who were held in hundreds of camps across Occupied Asia. We have to believe the very large number of Japanese medical personnel who repeatedly visited the camp, and who examined the prisoners and gave them injections, did so because they wished to cure the dysentery which was endemic to the camp. We have to believe the Japanese failure to distribute medicines to treat the illness they identified was perfectly proper and logical, or that the Japanese doctors were outrageously incompetent. We have to believe that even though official Japanese orders were issued by senior officers closely associated with Unit 731, no Unit 731 personnel visited the camp or had anything to do with the prisoners' health and wellbeing. We must also believe that all of the witnesses who gave statements concerning the tests that Japanese physicians performed on them – some of them invasive and demeaning tests, as well as multiple inoculations – were lying. We also must believe that Japanese officers who actually worked at Unit 731, such as Major Tomio Karasawa, who flatly stated Unit 731 researchers did conduct experiments on Allied POWs at Mukden, were also lying. We are asked to believe that when FBI Director J. Edgar Hoover asked for information about experiments on Allied POWs at Mukden from the Department of Defense in 1956, and was rebuffed, it was because the American government had absolutely nothing to hide. And so it goes on, with many more examples littering this story like so many half-buried corpses. The banal picture painted by the American and British governments simply does not reflect the evidence.

We can probably re-create what occurred at the Mukden Camp fairly accurately from the available evidence and testimonies, and in this author's opinion it's as fair an assessment as the fairy tale that has been promulgated by certain governments since the end of the war. At some point in 1942 a group of scientists at Unit 731 had begun to undertake research into the immunity of 'Anglo-Saxons' to particular diseases, primarily strains of dysentery. A Unit 731 research doctor, who was variously referred to by witnesses as 'Minato' or 'Minata', most probably headed the group and he was based in a known Unit 731 sub-station – the Mukden Military Hospital. This research would have been required as Japan was fast developing various lethal biological warfare weapons, and if they were going to use them against their major

Conclusion

enemies, the United States and Britain, testing them on captured Allied POWs made as much sense as using Chinese prisoners for tests when developing weapons to aid the Japanese takeover of China. The next problem for the Japanese was in finding the necessary human material for their research project.

The two main sources of English-speaking 'Anglo-Saxon' POWs that the Japanese possessed in 1942 were concentrated in a series of camps in the Philippines and in Singapore, the result of the massive American and British surrenders that had occurred during the early part of the year. An order was issued to assemble Allied POWs at Mukden, 350 miles south of the Unit 731 headquarters at Pingfan in Manchuria. We can make an educated guess as to why the majority of the prisoners who were assembled were Americans, rather than British, Australians or Dutch who had been captured in even greater numbers. It would make sense, from a medical point of view, to use American POWs as the main test subjects because the US Army contained examples of every regional type of Caucasian male due to the melting pot makeup of American society, thereby enabling doctors to compare and contrast a great number of different Caucasian types whose ancestors originally came from many different nations and geographical areas of Europe. This neatly explains the point of the detailed interviews conducted by the Japanese doctors at Mukden which probed the American prisoners' family backgrounds. It is also interesting to note that only 100 British and Australian prisoners were sent from Korean POW camps to Mukden. Why such a small number – why did the Japanese not just add another 100 Americans to their original shipment from the Philippines? The answer is again quite simple – the British and Australian prisoners represented for the Japanese the true 'Anglo-Saxons', historically and geographically, and this group would be less likely to demonstrate enormous differences in regional types of Caucasian found in the much more mixed American population of the period. At the time Britain was not a multicultural society like today, and Australians of the time also generally traced their ancestry back to Britain or Ireland. The British, who numbered roughly ten per cent of the total number of test subjects at Mukden, were the control group for the experiment – hence they did not perish when the Americans died literally like flies from some unknown dysentery-like disorder.

The Devil's Doctors

Some of the American prisoners were probably already infected with a strain of dysentery before they arrived at the temporary Mukden Camp – many of the veterans recalled examinations and inoculations while they were in transit from Pusan in Korea to Manchuria. Once the prisoners' were *in situ* at the new camp, an order was sent out from Kwantung Army HQ that dispatched a team of thirty-two Japanese doctors and medics from Unit 731 to the Mukden POW Camp. This group was most probably under the command of 'Dr. Minata'. Whether they came from the main Pingfan facility in the north of the province, or from the nearby Mukden Military Hospital, a known Unit 731 out-station, is unknown. But they were definitely Unit 731 personnel. The senior British officer at the camp, Major Robert Peaty, secretly noted the arrival of these personnel in his diary. Frank James recalled being forced to assist these self-same doctors with autopsies on American prisoners who had died from suspected dysentery, and this was corroborated by another entry made by Peaty in his diary. James also recalled in 1986 being interviewed in detail by the self-same Japanese doctors about his ancestry in 1943. Veterans James and Warren Whelchel both spoke of injections, anal examinations, and strange facial sprays on arrival at Mukden Camp, and similar events were also recounted by other veterans during the course of interviews.

From the available testimony it can be surmised that the selected prisoners were first subjected to a blood test. Following this, a group was deliberately infected with dysentery bacteria administered either as a facial spray, or given to them as a drink or within infected fruit. Many of the men subsequently developed severe dysentery and died. The Japanese team autopsied some of the bodies of the prisoners who had died from dysentery in order to assess the internal effects of the disease. This assertion is borne out by witness statements. Major Kawasawa stated in court in 1949 that Unit 731 doctors, specifically Dr. 'Minata', who was based with him at the Mukden Military Hospital close to the camp, was interested in testing the immunity of 'Anglo-Saxons' to disease. Another Unit 731 veteran, Tsuneji Shimada, said in 1985 that Dr. 'Minato' had deliberately infected American prisoners at the Mukden Camp with dysentery bacteria, and then performed blood tests on the prisoners, as well as autopsies at the camp. Many different witnesses stated the same thing, and only

Conclusion

two of them, Whelchel and James, appeared before the same Congressional subcommittee. The other statements were made at differing times, locations and circumstances, and by several different nationalities. Taken together, their statements paint a picture of the Japanese activities at Mukden Camp from four different time periods – Major Peaty secretly writing in 1943, Major Karasawa speaking on the stand in 1949, Warren Whelchel and Frank James under oath before Congress in 1982 and 1986 respectively, and Tsuneji Shimada speaking to reporters in 1985. We have the recurring name 'Minata' or 'Minato' that was mentioned by two Japanese witnesses fifty years apart, and we have the Japanese Army orders, signed by Lieutenant General Kajitsuka, chief doctor of the Kwantung Army and overseer of Unit 731, that ordered a specific number of medics to go to the Mukden Camp, and their arrival covertly recorded by witness Major Peaty in his diary.

The lack of documentary 'proof' in the form of Japanese documents which explicitly outlined a programme of experimentation upon Allied POWs at the Mukden Camp is not unreasonable considering the circumstances. Medical experiments on POWs constituted a war crime, and therefore such orders were carefully and obliquely worded, and the records carefully destroyed at the end of the war.

Each witness statement, and each piece of 'evidence' thus far presented, can be challenged and explained or individually dismissed with little difficulty. For this reason, we cannot conclude *beyond a reasonable doubt* that the Japanese conducted illegal human experiments at the Mukden Camp. More evidence needs to be found before such a concrete admission can become accepted historical truth. But when taken together, and looked at in a logical, linear order, the available evidence certainly casts *a reasonable doubt* over the official story of the purpose of the Mukden Camp. At the very least, the story of what actually happened to the American, British and Australian soldiers who were sent to Manchuria is far from settled, and as the remaining veterans pass away with their questions unanswered, and their beliefs and assertions often disparaged, much more needs to be done to discover the uncomfortable truth. Perhaps the most uncomfortable truth of all, and the real reason why we may never know the exact relationship between Unit 731 and the Mukden POWs is the undisputed fact that the United States military directly profited from the horrible deaths of tens of thousands of people at Pingfan and elsewhere, without a single voice of dissent being raised in moral outrage. That is the real reason behind the story of the Mukden prisoner-of-war camp, and the reason why even when it is quite obvious that something medically odd occurred at the camp, it remains extremely difficult to try and prove it.

Appendix A

British Prisoners-of-War, Mukden Camp[1]

Major Robert Peaty, Royal Army Ordnance Corps
Captain R.S. Horner, Federated Malay States Volunteer Force
Lieutenant A.L.N. Greig, Federated Malay States Volunteer Force
Second Lieutenant A.R. Griffin, Federated Malay States Volunteer Force
Staff-Sergeant Hanson, Royal Army Ordnance Corps
Sergeant Arnott, Royal Army Medical Corps
Sergeant Lee, 2nd Battalion, The Loyal Regiment
Sergeant Little, Royal Army Medical Corps
Sergeant Russell, Royal Army Medical Corps
Sergeant J. Roberts, Royal Army Medical Corps
Lance-Sergeant B.H. Farrant, (Unit unconfirmed)
Lance-Sergeant Gooby, 2nd Battalion, The Loyal Regiment (died of wounds from air raid 10/12/44)
Lance-Sergeant Reinhardt, (Unit unconfirmed)
Lance-Sergeant Woolham, (3854639), 2nd Battalion, The Loyal Regiment
Corporal Anger, Royal Army Medical Corps
Corporal Bee, (Unit unconfirmed)
Corporal Feeney, 2nd Battalion, The Loyal Regiment
Corporal Scott, (Unit unconfirmed)
Lance-Corporal Hick, Royal Army Medical Corps
Lance-Corporal Jolly, (Unit unconfirmed)
Lance-Corporal Porter, 2nd Battalion, The Loyal Regiment
Lance-Bombardier Scholl, 122 Field Regiment, Royal Artillery (killed in air raid 07/12/44)

Private Brierley, 2nd Battalion, The Loyal Regiment
Private Chapman, 2nd Battalion, The Loyal Regiment
Private Christie, 2nd Battalion, The Loyal Regiment
Private Crowley, (Unit unconfirmed)
Private Dickinson, 2nd Battalion, The Loyal Regiment
Private Duckworth, 2nd Battalion, The Loyal Regiment
Private Eccles, 2nd Battalion, The Loyal Regiment
Gunner Gunning, 122 Field Regiment, Royal Artillery
Private Hewitt, Royal Army Medical Corps
Private Heaton, 2nd Battalion, The Loyal Regiment
Private Hill, 2nd Battalion, The Loyal Regiment
Private Kyle, Royal Army Ordnance Corps
Private Mason, 2nd Battalion, The Loyal Regiment
Private Minshull, 2nd Battalion, The Loyal Regiment
Private Plummer, 2nd Battalion, The Loyal Regiment
Private Reeson, Royal Army Medical Corps
Private Rimmer, 2nd Battalion, The Loyal Regiment
Private Robinson, 2nd Battalion, The Loyal Regiment
Marine Rogers, Royal Marines
Private Scobie, (Unit unconfirmed)
Private Seales, Royal Army Medical Corps
Private Spencer, 2nd Battalion, The Loyal Regiment
Private Stanton, 2nd Battalion, The Loyal Regiment
Private Vaughan, Royal Army Medical Corps

Appendix B

Some Key Characters

Dr. Koji Ando
Head of Unit 731's Dalian Laboratory. Escaped prosecution for war crimes and was later a professor at Tokyo University Laboratory for Communicable Diseases, and Head, Central Laboratory for Experimental Animals.

General Baron Sadao Araki (1877–1966)
A charismatic right-wing army officer and political theorist, and one of the leaders of the radical wing of the army that invaded China. Minister of War 1931–36, and later Minister of Education, Araki was a close supporter of Shiro Ishii and Unit 731. Tried for war crimes, and sentenced to life imprisonment. Araki was released in 1955 and died in 1966 at the age of eighty-nine.

Chiang Kai-shek, Hon. GCB (1887–1975)
Leader of Nationalist China and Generalissimo of the Chinese armed forces since 1936. Chiang was instrumental in pressing the Allies to invade Burma in 1944. He was known also for his massive corruption and graft. Chiang and his formidable wife fled to Taiwan in 1949 when the communists took over the mainland.

Dr. Hideo Futagi
Head of Unit 731 vivisection team. Later a co-founder of the Green Cross Corporation in Japan.

HM Emperor Hirohito, Hon. KG (1901–1989)
The wartime Emperor of Japan, Hirohito and members of his family have been associated with war crimes by many historians.

Rehabilitated by the Japanese after the war, Hirohito lost his godlike position under the new constitution imposed upon Japan by General MacArthur, but is held in high regard in modern Japan today where he is known as the Emperor Showa.

Lieutenant General Dr. Shiro Ishii (1892–1959)
The microbiologist who created Unit 731. In 1940 Ishii was appointed Chief of the Bacteriological Warfare Section of the Kwantung Army. Between 1942 and 1945 he was Chief of the Medical Section of the Japanese 1st Army. Arrested by US occupation authorities in Japan in 1946, but given immunity from prosecution for war crimes in return for germ warfare data. Moved to Maryland, US, where he undertook research into bioweapons for the US Military. Died of throat cancer in Tokyo at the age of sixty-seven.

General Seishiro Itagaki (1885–1948)
Fought in the Russo-Japanese War 1904–05. Commanded a brigade in China 1927–29, and was later Chief of Intelligence Section of the Kwantung Army where he helped to plan the 1931 Mukden Incident. From 1937 to 1938 he commanded a division in China. Commanded Japanese 7th Area Army in Singapore and Malaya in 1945. Hanged as a war criminal at the age of sixty-three.

General Hyotaro Kimura (1888–1948)
Fought in Russia against the Bolsheviks in 1918–19 and served as military attaché to Germany. Commanded a division in China 1939–40 and was Chief of Staff of the Kwantung Army 1940–41. Vice Minister of War and member of the Supreme War Council. Later Commander-in-Chief, Burma Area Army 1944–45. Hanged as a war criminal at the age of sixty.

Lieutenant General Dr. Masaji Kitano (1894–1986)
Medical doctor, microbiologist and successor to Shiro Ishii as commander of Unit 731 in 1942. After the Japanese surrender in 1945 Kitano was detained in a prison camp in Shanghai before being repatriated back to Japan in January 1946. He never faced any war crimes charges. In Japan he worked for pharmaceutical company Green Cross, becoming the chief director in 1959. Kitano

APPENDIX B

was also on the Special Committee for Antarctic Research, as well as working for the Ministry of Education. He died in Tokyo at the age of ninety-one.

Colonel Dr. Chikahiko Koizumi (1884–1945)
Appointed Army Surgeon General in 1934, Koizumi was an early adherent of Shiro Ishii, and helped him to gain funding for his first human experimentation centre in Manchuria. Minister of Health 1941–45. Committed suicide 13 September 1945 to avoid a trial for war crimes.

Dr. Yoshisuke Murata
Commander of Unit 731 subordinate formation Unit 1644 in Nanjing, Murata escaped prosecution and later worked for the National Institute of Health.

Dr. Kozo Okamoto
Head of the Unit 731 pathology research team, Dr. Okamoto was later Dean, Faculty of Medicine at Kyoto University, and Dean, Faculty of Medicine at Kinki University.

Major General Dr. Shuniji Sato (1896–1977)
Commander of Unit 731 subordinate formation Unit 8604 in Guangzhou, China, 1941–43, then Chief of Medical Services, Japanese 5th Army 1943–45. Arrested by the Soviets in 1945 and arraigned before the Khabarovsk War Crimes Trial 1949. Sentenced to twenty years imprisonment. Died in Japan aged eighty-one.

Yoshio Shimozuka (b. 1923)
Served in Unit 731 as a medical orderly. One of the few veterans to confess that he was a member of the unit. Shimozuka has admitted to taking part in vivisection experiments on Chinese outside Harbin. In 1997 he gave testimony on behalf of 180 Chinese who were suing the Japanese government for compensation and an apology for the deaths of family members killed in experiments.

Dr. Tadao Sonoguchi
Unit 731 biological warfare development team. Later Vice-Principal, School of Hygiene of the Japan Self-Defense Forces, the nation's postwar military.

The Devil's Doctors

HIH Lieutenant-Colonel Prince Tsuneyoshi Takeda (1919–1992)
Emperor Hirohito's first cousin and the officer charged with executive responsibility for Unit 731 with Imperial General Headquarters, Tokyo. He visited Unit 731 and witnessed human experimentation. Became a commoner after the abolition of collateral branches of the Imperial Family in 1947. President of the Japan Olympic Committee 1962; he organised the 1964 Summer Olympics and the 1972 Winter Olympics and was a member of the International Olympic Committee 1967–81. He died suddenly of heart failure in 1992 aged eighty-three.

Dr. Hideo Tanaka
Unit 731 plague-carrying fleas team. After the war was appointed Dean, Faculty of Medicine, Osaka City University.

Field Marshal Count Hisaichi Terauchi (1879–1946)
Intimately involved with the Imperial Way faction of the army, career soldier Count Terauchi was the son of a former Japanese prime minister. He commanded the North China Area Army 1937–41 (with Unit 731 under command), and the 680,000 strong Southern Expeditionary Army Group 1941–45. Died of a stroke in a British POW camp in 1946 before standing trial for war crimes.

General Hideki Tojo (1884–1947)
Prime Minister of Japan and Minister of War 1941–44. He was also the driving force behind the appalling treatment of Allied prisoners-of-war and civilian internees. Hanged as a war criminal in 1947.

Appendix C

Japanese Army Chemical and Biological Warfare Units

Headquarters: Unit 731 (Togo Unit)
Location: Pingfang, Harbin, Manchukuo
Commander: Lieutenant General Shiro Ishii, 1934–42, then Major General Masaji Kitano, 1942–45

Sub-Units:

Unit 100
Location: Mokotan, Changchun, Manchukuo
Commander: Colonel Yujiro Wakamatsu

Unit 200
Location: Manchukuo

Unit 516 (Tsushogo Unit)
Location: Qigihar, Manchukuo

Unit 534
Location: Hailar, Manchukuo

Unit 773
Location: Songo, China

Unit Ei 1644
Location: Nanking (now Nanjing), China

Unit 2646 (or Unit 80)
Location: Hailar, Manchukuo

Unit 8604 (Nami Unit)
Location: Canton (now Guangzhou), China
Commander: Major General Shuniji Sato, 1941–43

Unit 9420 (Oka Unit)
Location: Tanpoi, Johor, Malaya & Singapore (with possible sub-units in Thailand)
Commander: Major General Kitagawa Masataka, 1942–45

Appendix D

Asia-Pacific War Timeline

1935
Autumn — Dr. Shiro Ishii established Unit 731 at Pingfan, Manchuria

1936
— Emperor Hirohito issues Imperial Decree expanding Unit 731
25 November — Japan signs the Anti-Comintern Pact with Germany

1937
7 July — Japan invades China
13 December — Start of the 'Rape of Nanking'

1939
May–August — Japanese and Soviet forces fight the Battle of Nomonhan on the Manchurian-Mongolian border and Japan is defeated
1 September — **Germany invades Poland**
3 September — **France, Britain and the Commonwealth declares war on Germany**

1940
22 June — **France falls to the Germans**
— Japan invades and occupies French Indochina
26 June — United States places an embargo on iron and steel imports to Japan
August — 'Unit 731' name first used by the Japanese

179

27 September	Japan signs the Tripartite Pact with Germany and Italy
	Plague-infested fleas dropped on Chinese city of Ningbo

1941

10 January	Thailand invades French Indochina
	Plague-infested fleas dropped on Chinese city of Changde
22 June	**Germany invades the Soviet Union**
26 July	United States places an oil embargo on Japan
7 December	**Japanese bomb Pearl Harbor, Wake Island, Midway Island and the Philippines**
8 December	**Japanese invade British Malaya, Thailand and Hong Kong**
9 December	China declares war on the Axis Powers
10 December	Japan sinks the British capital ships HMS *Prince of Wales* and HMS *Repulse* off Malaya and begins landings on the Philippines
14 December	**Japan invades Burma**
16 December	**Japan invades Borneo**
20 December	Japan attacks the Netherlands East Indies
24 December	Japan occupies Wake Island after a bitter battle with US forces
25 December	**Hong Kong surrenders to the Japanese**

1942

3 February	Japanese forces begin landing in the Netherlands East Indies
	Japanese aircraft attack Port Moresby, New Guinea
15 February	**British forces surrender to the Japanese in Singapore**
	Japanese aircraft attack Darwin in Australia
	Unit 9420 established in Singapore
27 February	Japanese Navy wins the Battle of the Java Sea
8 March	Japanese invade New Guinea
6 April	Japanese invade the Admiralty and British Solomon Islands

Appendix D

9 April	US forces in the Bataan Peninsula, Philippines, surrender to the Japanese
18 April	The Doolittle Raid is launched on Tokyo
1 May	Japanese forces capture Mandalay, Burma
6 May	US forces on Corregidor Island, Philippines, surrender to the Japanese
7 May	Battle of the Coral Sea
23 May	British withdrawal from Burma completed
4 June	Japanese attack Midway Island
6 June	Japanese invade the Aleutian Islands
	US Navy is victorious at The Battle of Midway
7 August	US forces land on Guadalcanal in the British Solomon Islands
9 August	Japanese Navy victorious at the Battle of Savo Island
12 August	Japanese land at Buna, New Guinea
18 September	Australian forces begin advancing down the Kokoda Trail, New Guinea
11–12 October	Japanese Navy defeated at the Battle of Cape Esperance
17 October	British forces advance into the Arakan, Burma
26 October	Japanese Navy victorious at the Battle of Santa Cruz
11 November	Allied POWs arrive at the temporary Mukden Camp

1943

2 February	**Soviet Union wins the Battle of Stalingrad**
13 February	British launch the first Chindit expedition into Burma
	Allied POWs moved to new Mukden Camp
2 March	Battle of the Bismarck Sea
20 June	US forces invade New Georgia
3 September	**Allied forces land in Italy**
20 November	US forces land on Tarawa

1944

31 January	US forces land in the Marshall Islands
2 March	British launch second Chindit expedition into Burma

15 March	Japanese invade India at Imphal and Kohima
22 April	US forces land at Hollandia, New Guinea
31 May	Japanese begin withdrawing from Kohima
4 June	**Allied forces capture Rome**
6 June	**D-Day landings in Normandy, France**
15 June	US forces land on Saipan
19 June	Commencement of the Battle of the Philippine Sea
18 July	Japanese forces begin withdrawing from Imphal
15 September	US forces land on Peleliu
20 October	US forces land on Leyte, Philippines
24–25 October	Battle of Leyte Gulf
12 November	Hoten Branch Camp No. 1 established for 246 Allied officers and men
	British 14th Army enters Burma
1 December	Hoten Branch Camp No. 2 established for 34 Allied senior officers
7 December	Mukden Camp bombed by the Americans
21 December	Mukden Camp bombed by the Americans

1945

9 January	US forces land on Luzon, Philippines
11 January	British forces cross the Irrawaddy River, Burma
19 February	US forces land on Iwo Jima
2 March	British forces capture Meiktila, Burma
20 March	British forces capture Mandalay, Burma
1 April	US forces land on Okinawa
12 April	**President Roosevelt dies**
29 April	134 new POWs arrive at Mukden Camp
30 April	**Hitler dies in Berlin**
3 May	British forces enter Rangoon, Burma
8 May	**Germany surrenders**
20 May	Hoten Branch Camp No. 1 closed and POWs sent to Mukden Camp
26 July	**Churchill resigns as British Prime Minister**
6 August	Atomic bomb dropped on Hiroshima, Japan – POWs beaten at Mukden
8 August	Soviet Union declares war on Japan and invades Manchuria

Appendix D

9 August	Atomic bomb dropped on Nagasaki, Japan
15 August	Japan announces its surrender
16 August	OSS team parachutes into Mukden Camp
20 August	Mukden Camp liberated by Soviet 6th Guards Tank Army
26 August	Soviet invasion of Manchuria complete
21 August–7 September	Aerial evacuations of prisoners from Mukden Camp
29 August	POW Recovery Team 1 arrives at Mukden Camp
2 September	Formal surrender of Japan
10–11 September	Mukden POWs leave for Dalian by train
19 September	Mukden Camp abandoned

Notes

Chapter 1: The Seeds of Death
1. Daniel Barenblatt, *A Plague Upon Humanity: The Secret Genocide of Axis Japan's Germ Warfare Operation* (London; Souvenir Press, 2006), 5
2. Hal Gold, *Unit 731 Testimony* (North Clarendon, VT; Tuttle Publishing, 1996), 23
3. Daniel Barenblatt, *A Plague Upon Humanity: The Secret Genocide of Axis Japan's Germ Warfare Operation* (London; Souvenir Press, 2006), 7
4. Hal Gold, *Unit 731 Testimony* (North Clarendon, VT; Tuttle Publishing, 1996), 23
5. The treaties signed in London and Washington in 1930 also meant that Britain's Royal Navy would no longer be the largest in the world, and in order to achieve parity of numbers with the United States Navy the Admiralty actually had to scrap some British ships. America became an equal partner with Britain in ruling Asia and the Pacific.
6. Daniel Barenblatt, *A Plague Upon Humanity: The Secret Genocide of Axis Japan's Germ Warfare Operation* (London; Souvenir Press, 2006), 18
7. Hal Gold, *Unit 731 Testimony* (North Clarendon, VT; Tuttle Publishing, 1996), 30
8. Mark Felton, *Japan's Gestapo: Murder, Mayhem and Torture in Wartime Asia* (Barnsley; Pen & Sword Books, 2009), 28
9. Daniel Barenblatt, *A Plague Upon Humanity: The Secret Genocide of Axis Japan's Germ Warfare Operation* (London; Souvenir Press, 2006), 17

Chapter 2: Paris of the Orient
1. Hal Gold, *Unit 731 Testimony* (North Clarendon, VT; Tuttle Publishing, 1996), 38
2. Sheldon H. Harris, *Factories of Death: Japanese Biological Warfare 1944–5 and the American Cover-up* (New York; Routledge, 1994), 32

NOTES

3. Ibid: 33
4. Daniel Barenblatt, *A Plague Upon Humanity: The Secret Genocide of Axis Japan's Germ Warfare Operation* (London; Souvenir Press, 2006), 29
5. Ibid: 33–1
6. Sheldon H. Harris, *Factories of Death: Japanese Biological Warfare 1944–5 and the American Cover-up* (New York; Routledge, 1994), 34
7. Hal Gold, *Unit 731 Testimony* (North Clarendon, VT; Tuttle Publishing, 1996), 40
8. Daniel Barenblatt, *A Plague Upon Humanity: The Secret Genocide of Axis Japan's Germ Warfare Operation* (London; Souvenir Press, 2006), 44–3
9. Sheldon H. Harris, *Factories of Death: Japanese Biological Warfare 1944–5 and the American Cover-up* (New York; Routledge, 1994), 34
10. Mark Felton, *Japan's Gestapo: Murder, Mayhem and Torture in Wartime Asia* (Barnsley; Pen & Sword Books, 2009), 123
11. Daniel Barenblatt, *A Plague Upon Humanity: The Secret Genocide of Axis Japan's Germ Warfare Operation* (London; Souvenir Press, 2006), 44

Chapter 3: Blood Harvest

1. Sheldon H. Harris, *Factories of Death: Japanese Biological Warfare 1944–5 and the American Cover-up* (New York; Routledge, 1994), 42
2. *Doctors of Depravity* by Christopher Hudson, *Daily Mail*, 2 March 2007
3. *Archives give up secrets of Japan's Unit 731*, *China Daily*, 3 August 2005
4. Mark Felton, *Japan's Gestapo: Murder, Mayhem and Torture in Wartime Asia* (Barnsley; Pen & Sword Books, 2009), 124
5. *Unmasking Horror – A special report: Japan Confronting Gruesome War Atrocity* by Nicholas D. Kristof, *New York Times*, 17 March 1995
6. *Doctors of Depravity* by Christopher Hudson, *Daily Mail*, 2 March 2007
7. Ibid.
8. Ibid.
9. *Materials on the Trial of Former Servicemen of the Japanese Army Charged with Manufacturing and Employing Bacteriological Weapons* (Moscow; Foreign Languages Publishing House, 1950)
10. *Unmasking Horror – A special report: Japan Confronting Gruesome War Atrocity* by Nicholas D. Kristof, *New York Times*, 17 March 1995

Chapter 4: The Camp

1. Sheldon H. Harris, *Factories of Death* (New York; Routledge, 2002), 124
2. Ibid: 124

3. Mark Felton, *The Coolie Generals: Britain's Far Eastern Military Leaders in Japanese Captivity* (Barnsley; Pen & Sword Books, 2006), 118
4. Ibid: 118
5. Arthur Percival, *The War in Malaya* (London; Eyre & Spottiswoode, 1949), 312
6. *Diary of Major Robert Peaty*, Cat. No. 6377; Private Papers of Major R. Peaty, Imperial War Museum, London
7. *Report by Major Stanley Hankins*, Record Group 389, Stack 290, Row 34, Compartment 13, Entry 360A, Box 2127, National Archives and Records Administration (NARA), Washington D.C., courtesy of: Mukden Prisoner of War Remembrance Society
8. Linda Goetz Holmes, *Unjust Enrichment: How Japan's Companies Built Postwar Fortunes Using American POWs* (Mechanicsburg, PA; Stackpole Books, 2001)
9. Ibid.
10. The National Archives (TNA); Public Record Office (PRO) CO968/98/6, *Despatch on Surrender of Hong Kong, Sir Mark Young to Secretary of State for the Colonies*; 12 September 1945
11. Stella Dong, *Shanghai: The Rise and Fall of a Decadent City* (New York; William Morrow, Perennial, 2001), 272–77
12. Lord Russell of Liverpool, *The Knights of Bushido: A Short History of Japanese War Crimes* (London; Greenhill Books, 2002), 85
13. Ibid: 152
14. *Report by Major Mark Herbst*; Record Group 389, Stack 290, Row 34, Compartment 13, Entry 360A, Box 2127, National Archives and Records Administration (NARA), Washington D.C., courtesy of: Mukden Prisoner of War Remembrance Society
15. Lord Russell of Liverpool, *The Knights of Bushido: A Short History of Japanese War Crimes* (London; Greenhill Books, 2002), 159
16. *Report by Major Stanley Hankins*, Record Group 389, Stack 290, Row 34, Compartment 13, Entry 360A, Box 2127, National Archives and Records Administration (NARA), Washington D.C., courtesy of: Mukden Prisoner of War Remembrance Society
17. *Report by Major Mark Herbst*, Record Group 389, Stack 290, Row 34, Compartment 13, Entry 360A, Box 2127, National Archives and Records Administration (NARA), Washington D.C., courtesy of: Mukden Prisoner of War Remembrance Society
18. *Diary of Major Robert Peaty*, Cat. No. 6377; Private Papers of Major R. Peaty, Imperial War Museum, London
19. Ibid.
20. Ibid.

Notes

21. Lord Russell of Liverpool, *The Knights of Bushido: A Short History of Japanese War Crimes* (London; Greenhill Books, 2002), 151
22. Ibid: 84
23. Ibid: 159
24. *Report by Major Mark Herbst*; Record Group 389, Stack 290, Row 34, Compartment 13, Entry 360A, Box 2127, National Archives and Records Administration (NARA), Washington D.C., courtesy of: Mukden Prisoner of War Remembrance Society
25. Ibid.
26. Ibid.
27. Lord Russell of Liverpool, *The Knights of Bushido: A Short History of Japanese War Crimes* (London, Greenhill Books, 2002), 88
28. Gavan Daws, *Prisoners of the Japanese: POWs of the Second World War in the Pacific* (London: Pocket Books, 2007), 205
29. Lord Russell of Liverpool, *The Knights of Bushido: A Short History of Japanese War Crimes* (London, Greenhill Books, 2002), 156

Chapter 5: Forced Labour

1. *Report by Major Stanley Hankins*, Record Group 389, Stack 290, Row 34, Compartment 13, Entry 360A, Box 2127, National Archives and Records Administration (NARA), Washington D.C., courtesy of: Mukden Prisoner of War Remembrance Society
2. Raymond Lamont-Brown, *Kempeitai: Japan's Dreaded Military Police* (Sutton Publishing, 1998), 125
3. *Diary of Major Robert Peaty*, Cat. No. 6377, Private Papers of Major R. Peaty, Imperial War Museum, London
4. *Report by Major Stanley Hankins*, Record Group 389, Stack 290, Row 34, Compartment 13, Entry 360A, Box 2127, National Archives and Records Administration (NARA), Washington D.C., courtesy of: Mukden Prisoner of War Remembrance Society
5. Ibid.
6. *Diary of Major Robert Peaty*, Cat. No. 6377, Private Papers of Major R. Peaty, Imperial War Museum, London
7. *Report by Major Stanley Hankins*, Record Group 389, Stack 290, Row 34, Compartment 13, Entry 360A, Box 2127, National Archives and Records Administration (NARA), Washington D.C., courtesy of: Mukden Prisoner of War Remembrance Society
8. *Diary of Major Robert Peaty*, Cat. No. 6377, Private Papers of Major R. Peaty, Imperial War Museum, London
9. *Laden, Fevered, Starved – The POWs of Sandakan, North Borneo, 1945*, Commonwealth Department of Veterans' Affairs, http://www.dva.gov.au, accessed 6 August 2008

10. Lord Russell of Liverpool, *The Knights of Bushido: A Short History of Japanese War Crimes* (London; Greenhill Books, 2002), 177
11. Ibid: 179
12. Ibid: 179
13. Ibid: 86
14. Gavan Daws, *Prisoners of the Japanese: POWs of the Second World War* (London; Pocket Books, 1994), 149
15. Ibid: 149
16. Ibid: 149
17. Ibid: 150
18. Chester M. Briggs, Jr., *Behind the Barbed Wire: Memoirs of a World War II US Marine Captured in North China in 1941 and Imprisoned by the Japanese until 1945* (McFarland & Company, 1994)
19. *Diary of Major Robert Peaty*, Cat. No. 6377, Private Papers of Major R. Peaty, Imperial War Museum, London
20. Ibid.
21. Gavan Daws, *Prisoners of the Japanese: POWs of the Second World War* (London; Pocket Books, 1994), 158

Chapter 6: Guinea Pigs

1. *Diary of Major Robert Peaty*, Cat. No. 6377, Private Papers of Major R. Peaty, Imperial War Museum, London
2. Hal Gold, *Unit 731 Testimony: Japan's Wartime Human Experimentation Program* (North Clarendon, VT; Tuttle Publishing, 1996), 172
3. Ibid: 240
4. Ibid: 242–41
5. *Diary of Major Robert Peaty*, Cat. No. 6377, Private Papers of Major R. Peaty, Imperial War Museum, London
6. Ibid.
7. Ibid.
8. Ibid.
9. Ibid.
10. Sheldon H. Harris, *Factories of Death* (New York; Routledge, 2002), 126
11. *Diary of Major Robert Peaty*, Cat. No. 6377, Private Papers of Major R. Peaty, Imperial War Museum, London
12. Ibid.
13. Ibid.
14. Ibid.
15. Ibid.
16. Ibid.
17. Sheldon H. Harris, *Factories of Death* (New York; Routledge, 2002), 126

NOTES

18. *Diary of Major Robert Peaty*, Cat. No. 6377, Private Papers of Major R. Peaty, Imperial War Museum, London
19. *A Historical and Ethical Examination of the Khabarovsk War Crimes Trial* by B.G. Yudin, 21 February 2008, *International Portal for the Humanities*, www.zpu-journal.ru, accessed 2 February 2010
20. Anon., *Materials of the Trial of Former Servicemen of the Japanese Army Accused in Manufacture and Use of Biological Weapons* (Moscow; State Publishing House of Political Literature, 1950 (in Russian)), 265
21. *Beijing Bright Daily*, 1 June 1994
22. Linda Goetz Holmes, *Unjust Enrichment: How Japan's Companies Built Postwar Fortunes Using American POWs* (Mechanicsburg, PA: Stackpole Books, 2001)
23. *Beijing Bright Daily*, 1 June 1994
24. Sheldon H. Harris, *Factories of Death* (New York; Routledge, 2002), 120
25. Ibid: 111–18
26. Ibid: 118
27. Ibid: 117
28. Linda Goetz Holmes, *Unjust Enrichment: How Japan's Companies Built Postwar Fortunes Using American POWs* (Mechanicsburg, PA: Stackpole Books, 2001)
29. Sheldon H. Harris, *Factories of Death* (New York; Routledge, 2002), 120
30. *Diary of Major Robert Peaty*, Cat. No. 6377, Private Papers of Major R. Peaty, Imperial War Museum, London
31. Linda Goetz Holmes, *Unjust Enrichment: How Japan's Companies Built Postwar Fortunes Using American POWs* (Mechanicsburg, PA: Stackpole Books, 2001)
32. Ibid.
33. Ibid.
34. Ibid.
35. Daniel Barenblatt, *A Plague Upon Humanity: The Secret Genocide of Axis Japan's Germ Warfare Operation* (New York; Souvenir Press, 2004), 180
36. Sheldon H. Harris, *Factories of Death* (New York; Routledge, 2002), 120
37. Ibid: 120
38. Ibid: 120
39. Anon., *Materials of the Trial of Former Servicemen of the Japanese Army Accused in Manufacture and Use of Biological Weapons* (Moscow; State Publishing House of Political Literature, 1950 (in Russian)), 265
40. Ibid: 115

Chapter 7: Precedents and Paper Trails

1. Daniel Barenblatt, *A Plague Upon Humanity: The Secret Genocide of Axis Japan's Germ Warfare Operation* (New York; Souvenir Press, 2004), 181
2. Sheldon H. Harris, *Factories of Death* (New York; Routledge, 2002), 121
3. Ibid: 121
4. Ibid: 122
5. Ibid: 122
6. 'National Affairs: Back from the Grave', *TIME*, 10 September 1945
7. Daniel Barenblatt, *A Plague Upon Humanity: The Secret Genocide of Axis Japan's Germ Warfare Operation* (New York; Souvenir Press, 2004), 181
8. 'National Affairs: Back from the Grave', *TIME*, 10 September 1945
9. 'War Crimes: For God's Sake!', *TIME*, 16 February 1948
10. 'National Affairs: Back from the Grave', *TIME*, 10 September 1945
11. 'A quiet honesty records a World War II atrocity' by Thomas Easton, *The Baltimore Sun*, 28 May 1995
12. Daniel Barenblatt, *A Plague Upon Humanity: The Secret Genocide of Axis Japan's Germ Warfare Operation* (New York; Souvenir Press, 2004), 183
13. *Diary of Major Robert Peaty*, Cat. No. 6377, Private Papers of Major R. Peaty, Imperial War Museum, London
14. Ibid.
15. Ibid.
16. Ibid.
17. Ibid.

Chapter 8: Flamingo

1. *Unmasking Horror – A special report: Japan Confronting Gruesome War Atrocity* by Nicholas D. Kristof, *New York Times*, 17 March 1995
2. Hal Gold, *Unit 731 Testimony: Japan's Wartime Human Experimentation Program* (North Clarendon, VT; Tuttle Publishing, 1996), 161–70
3. Ibid: 181
4.: 243
5. *Beijing Bright Daily*, 1 June 1994
6. Detachment 101 (Burma), Detachment 202 (China), Detachment 303 (New Delhi, India), Detachment 505 (Calcutta, India)
7. Daniel Barenblatt, *A Plague Upon Humanity: The Secret Genocide of Axis Japan's Germ Warfare Operation* (New York; Souvenir Press, 2004), 177
8. Ibid: 177

NOTES

9. Lord Russell of Liverpool, *The Knights of Bushido: A Short History of Japanese War Crimes* (London; Greenhill Books, 2002), 116
10. *War Ministry to Commanding General of Military Police, 1 August 1944*, Document No. 2710, Record Group 238, Box 2015, National Archives and Records Administration (NARA), Washington D.C.
11. Ibid.
12. Imperial Japanese Army, Box 263, Exhibit 1978, Document No. 1114-B: *Regarding the outline for the disposal of Prisoners of War according to the change of situation, a notification, Army-Asia-Secret No. 2257, by the Vice War Minister*, 11 March 1945, MacMillan Brown Library, University of Canterbury, Christchurch, New Zealand
13. Ibid.
14. *Chief Prisoner of War Camps Tokyo to Chief of Staff, Taiwan Army, 20 August 1945*, Document No. 2697, Record Group 238, Box 2011, National Archives and Records Administration (NARA), Washington D.C.
15. Ibid.
16. Ibid: 177

Chapter 9: Reaping the Whirlwind

1. Hal Gold, *Unit 731 Testimony: Japan's Wartime Human Experimentation Program* (North Clarendon, VT; Tuttle Publishing, 1996), 99–7
2. *Japanese Biological Warfare Intelligence, Inter-Service Sub-Committee on Biological Warfare, 16 January 1946*, The National Archives (Public Record Office), WO188/659
3. Ibid: 16 January 1946
4. Hal Gold, *Unit 731 Testimony: Japan's Wartime Human Experimentation Program* (North Clarendon, VT; Tuttle Publishing, 1996), 97
5. *Report on Scientific Intelligence Survey in Japan – September and October 1945, Volume V, Biological Warfare*. (GHQ, US Army Forces, Pacific, Scientific and Technical Section, 1 November 1945), annex to: *Japanese Biological Warfare Intelligence, Inter-Service Sub-Committee on Biological Warfare, 16 January 1946*, The National Archives (Public Record Office), WO188/659
6. Ibid, 1 November 1945
7. Ibid, 1 November 1945
8. *Inter-Service Sub-Committee on Biological Warfare, Minutes of a Meeting*, 10 May 1946, The National Archives (Public Record Office), WO188/659
9. Ibid: 10 May 1946
10. Daniel Barenblatt, *A Plague Upon Humanity: The Secret Genocide of Axis Japan's Germ Warfare Operation* (New York; Souvenir Press, 2004), 207

11. *Inter-Service Sub-Committee on Biological Warfare, Minutes of a Meeting*, 10 May 1946, The National Archives (Public Record Office), WO188/659
12. Sheldon H. Harris, *Factories of Death* (New York; Routledge, 2002), 114
13. Ibid: 115
14. Ibid: 115
15. Ibid: 115
16. Hal Gold, *Unit 731 Testimony: Japan's Wartime Human Experimentation Program* (North Clarendon, VT; Tuttle Publishing, 1996), 108
17. Ibid: 103
18. Daniel Barenblatt, *A Plague Upon Humanity: The Secret Genocide of Axis Japan's Germ Warfare Operation* (New York; Souvenir Press, 2004), 208
19. *Inter-Service Sub-Committee on Biological Warfare, Minutes of a Meeting*, 10 May 1946, The National Archives (Public Record Office), WO188/659
20. Daniel Barenblatt, *A Plague Upon Humanity: The Secret Genocide of Axis Japan's Germ Warfare Operation* (New York; Souvenir Press, 2004), 210
21. Ibid: 211
22. Ibid: 212
23. Hal Gold, *Unit 731 Testimony: Japan's Wartime Human Experimentation Program* (North Clarendon, VT; Tuttle Publishing, 1996), 107
24. Ibid: 107
25. Ibid: 110
26. Ibid: 111
27. Ibid: 111
28. Daniel Barenblatt, *A Plague Upon Humanity: The Secret Genocide of Axis Japan's Germ Warfare Operation* (New York; Souvenir Press, 2004), 217
29. Hal Gold, *Unit 731 Testimony: Japan's Wartime Human Experimentation Program* (North Clarendon, VT; Tuttle Publishing, 1996), 115
30. *Inter-Service Sub-Committee on Biological Warfare, Minutes of a Meeting*, The National Archives (Public Record Office), WO188/660
31. Hal Gold, *Unit 731 Testimony: Japan's Wartime Human Experimentation Program* (North Clarendon, VT; Tuttle Publishing, 1996), 107
32. *Materials on the Trial of Former Servicemen of the Japanese Army Charged with Manufacturing and Employing Bacteriological Weapons* (Moscow; Foreign Languages Publishing House, 1950)
33. Daniel Barenblatt, *A Plague Upon Humanity: The Secret Genocide of Axis Japan's Germ Warfare Operation* (New York; Souvenir Press, 2004), 223
34. See: Sheldon H. Harris, *Factories of Death: Japanese Biological Warfare 1944–5 and the American Cover-up* (New York; Routledge, 1994)

NOTES

Chapter 10: Operation 'PX'

1. Mark Felton, *The Fujita Plan: Japanese Attacks on the United States and Australia during the Second World War* (Barnsley; Pen & Sword Books, 2006), 141–43
2. A balloon gondola and its payload can be viewed at the Canadian Military Museum in Ottawa.
3. Mark Felton, *The Fujita Plan: Japanese Attacks on the United States and Australia during the Second World War* (Barnsley; Pen & Sword Books, 2006), 194
4. Ibid: 194
5. *War Cabinet Bacteriological Warfare Committee: correspondence*, The National Archives (Public Record Office), WO188/654
6. Ibid.
7. Ibid.
8. Henry Sakaida, Gary Nila & Koji Takaki, *I-400: Japan's Secret Panama Canal Strike Submarine* (Hikoki Publications, 2006)
9. Data derived from Bob Hackett & Sander Kingsepp's *'Sensuikan'*, http://www.combinedfleet.com/sensuikan.htm
10. Hal Gold, *Unit 731 Testimony: Japan's Wartime Human Experimentation Program* (Tuttle Publishing, 1996), 89
11. Ibid: 91

Chapter 11: Dark Harvest

1. *Porton Down – The Terrible Secret*, Global-Elite.org, http://www.rense.com/general39/secret.htm; accessed 13 April 2011
2. Wikipedia; accessed 21 March 2011
3. *Porton Down – The Terrible Secret*, Global-Elite.org, http://www.rense.com/general39/secret.htm; accessed 13 April 2011
4. Ibid.
5. Wikipedia; accessed 21 March 2011

Appendix A: British Prisoners-of-War, Mukden Camp

1. This information is not exhaustive, but is instead a list of *confirmed* British POWs who were transported to Mukden Camp in late 1942. It is drawn from Major Robert Peaty's diary and Red Army evacuation rosters. It excludes the 'Senior Officers Party', and the other ranks soldiers that were batmen and cooks with this party. (Sources: www.mansell.com and the *Diary of Major Robert Peaty*, Cat. No. 6377, Private Papers of Major R. Peaty, Imperial War Museum, London)

Index

Araki, Gen. Sadao, 16
Ariizumi, Capt. Tatsunosuke, 154
Ashurst, Col. William, 51
Australian Army:
  Australian Army Medical Corps, 47
  Australian Artillery, 56
  Australian Pioneer Corps, 52
Autumn Storm (1945), Operation, 120–4

Bataan Death March (1942), 41
Batu Lintang Prison Camp, 48, 56–7, 60–1
Bochsel, Chief Warrant Officer A.A., 54
Botterill, Pvt. Keith, 68
Bottomley, Air Vice Marshal Sir Norman, 129
Braddon, Gnr. Russell, 56
Brennan, Capt. Desmond, 47, 58, 96, 116
British Army:
  Royal Army Ordnance Corps, 45
  Royal Artillery, 43, 105
  The Loyal Regiment (North Lancashire), 43, 105
Burma-Thailand Railway, 51, 57, 59–60, 68–9

Campbell, Art, 92
Changi Prison Camp (Singapore), 43, 64
Chastain, Sgt. Joseph, 66
Chiang Kai-shek, Generalissimo, 17
Churchill, Winston, 122

Davis, W. Wesley, 91
Donovan, Lt.-Col. James, 110

Eight Mile Prison Camp (North Borneo), 56–7
Endo, Lt.-Gen. Saburo, 26
Eno, Capt. Yoshio, 154–5

Fujita, Chief Warrant Officer Nobuo, 146
Fukian Maru (transport ship), 43, 45

Index

Geneva Convention (1925), 10–11, 18
Gottlieb, Capt. Robert, 100, 103

Hague Convention (1899), 11
Hamaguchi, Osachi, 16
Hankins, Maj. Stanley, 45–6, 49, 55, 65, 81
Haroekoe Prison Camp (Moluccas), 52–4, 57, 61
Hatcher, Dr. John, 101
Hattori, Col. Takushiro, 155
Herbst, Capt. Mark, 47, 54–5, 58–9, 81, 96
Hirazakura, Lt. Zensaku, 141
Hirohito, Emperor, 13, 27–8, 128, 136
Hitler, Adolf, 18
Holland, William, 104
Hoover, J. Edgar, 94–5, 121, 166
Hoshijima, Capt. Susumi, 48–9, 67–8

Imperial Japanese Army:
  Anti-Epidemic Water Supply & Purification Bureau, 23, 33
  Kempeitai Military Police, 17, 20, 28, 32–3, 44, 64
  Kwantung Army, 17–18, 121, 123
  Togo Unit, 22–7, 28
  Tokyo Army Medical College, 18
  Unit 731 *see* Unit 731
International Military Tribunal for the Far East, 132–3
Ishii, Lt.-Gen. Shiro, 6, 8, 10–14, 16–20, 22–7, 31, 34, 36–7, 58–9, 86–8, 95, 107, 120–1, 124–5, 131–2, 142, 145–6, 150–1, 155, 163
Ishihara, Isamu, 69–70
Ishiwara, Lt.-Col. Kenji, 17, 19
Ishiyama, Dr. Fumio, 109
Itagaki, Col. Seishiro, 17

James, Frank, 89–91, 93–4, 98, 168, 169
Japanese Army *see* Imperial Japanese Army
Japan:
  Imperial Way Faction, 15–16, 19
  Meiji Restoration (1868), 12
  Rise of Militarism, 16–17

Kajitsuka, Lt.-Gen. Ryuji, 86–7, 94, 141
Karasawa, Maj. Tomio, 26, 87, 93, 132, 138, 141–2, 166
Keenan, Joseph, 133
Kelleher, James, 95
Kempeitai Military Police *see* Imperial Japanese Army
Keschner, Capt. Harold, 103–104
Khabarovsk War Crimes Trial (1949), 86–7, 132, 140–2
Kido, Fumio, 110
Kikuchi, Col. Hitoshi, 133
Kikuchi, Corp. Norimitsu, 141
Kitagawa, Maj.-Gen. Masataka, 35
Kitano, Dr. Masaji, 142
Koizumi, Col. Chikahiko, 18
Koshi, Sadao, 115
Kurushima, Pvt. Yuji, 141

Kusaba, Maj.-Gen. Sueyoshi, 147
Kwarenko Prison Camp (Manchuria), 67

Lamar, Maj. Robert, 110
League of Nations, 18–19
Leith, Corp. Hal, 110

MacArthur, Gen. Douglas, 127–8, 130–1, 133–4, 137, 163
Maddison, Leading Aircraftman Ronald, 160–2
Makassar Prison Camp, 63, 68
Manchuria:
  Japanese takeover, 15
  Manchukuo, 19
  Mukden Incident, 17–18
  South Manchurian Railway, 17, 124
  White Russians, 21–2
  Zhongma Fortress, 21–4
Matsuda, Col. Genji, 49
Meringolo, Seaman 1st Class Ferdinand, 66
Mikasa, Prince, 39
Mitomo, Senior Sgt. Kazuo, 141
Morishita, Kiyohito, 116
Mukden Military Hospital, 6, 46, 58–9, 82, 94, 166, 168
Mukden Prison Camp (Manchuria):
  Administration, 46–7
  Air raids, 105–106
  Arrival of POWs, 46
  Autopsies, 88–9
  Clothing, 62–3
  Death rate, 57–8, 82–3
  Evacuation, 111–12
  Food, 54–6
  Guards, 48
  Layout, 50, 53
  Liberation, 110–11
  Location, 46
  Mail, 63–4
  Medical examinations, 84
  Medical facilities, 58–9, 78–80
  Mitsubishi factories, 49–50, 72
  POW pay, 63
  Punishments, 65–7
  Recreation, 63
  Relocation of camp, 71–2
  Transportation of POWs, 41–5
  Vaccinations, 79, 88–9
  Washing facilities, 54
  Weather, 47
Murray, Prof. G.D., 150

Nagata, Maj.-Gen. Tetsuru, 16–17
Nagayama, Dr. Saburo, 85
Naito, Lt.-Col. Ryoichi, 126–8, 130–1, 139
Nakanishi, Sadayoshi, 119
Nishi, Lt.-Col. Toshihide, 141

Onoue, Maj. Masao, 141
Opium War (China), 15
Ota, Col. Kiyoshi, 133
Ozawa, Vice Admiral Jisaburo, 154–5

Paliotti, Corp. Victor, 66
Peaty, Maj. Robert, 1, 45–7, 54–7, 62, 64–5, 70–1, 79, 81–3, 85, 88–9, 112, 168

Index

Percival, Lt.-Gen. Arthur, 43, 59, 65, 67, 75, 105
Ponczha, Sgt. Edward, 108
Porton Down (Defence Science and Technology Laboratory), 159–64
Prevuzniak, Sgt. Andrew, 54

River Valley Road Prison Camp 17 (Japan), 64
Rodriguez, Gregory, 91–2
Roling, B.V.A., 142

Sandakan Prison Camps (Borneo), 48–9, 67–8
Sanders, Col. Murray, 126–8
Sato, Maj.-Gen. Shinuji, 141
Schreiner, Pvt. Sigmund, 41–2, 80
Shimada, Tsuneji, 94
Shinagawa POW Hospital (Japan), 102–104, 132
Sian Prison Camp (Manchuria), 72–3
Sonei, Capt. Kenichi, 48
Songkrei Prison Camp (Thailand), 52
Springer, Dr. R., 53–4, 61
Stalin, Josef, 12
Starz, Sgt. Edward, 110
Suga, Lt.-Col. Tatsuji, 48
Sun Yat-sen, 14

Takahashi, Korekiyu, 13–14
Takahashi, Lt.-Gen. Takaatsu, 141
Tanjong Maru (transport ship), 43–4
Tan Toey Barracks Prison Camp (Amboina), 52, 56

Thomas, Sir Shenton, 73
Thompson, Col. Arvo, 135, 139
Tjideng Ghetto (Batavia), 48
Tojo, Gen. Hideki, 18, 39, 72
Tokada, Capt. Hisikichi, 103–104
Totori Maru (transport ship), 41–2, 45
Truman, Harry S., 121

Umezu, Gen. Yoshijiro, 85, 94, 155–7
Unit 731:
 Associated units, 34–5
 Biological Warfare attacks, 37
 Caucasian prisoners, 113–16
 Divisions, 33
 Evacuation, 124–5
 Experiments, 33–4, 36–8, 77–8, 86–8
 Imperial Family, 136–7
 Guards, 30
 Layout, 30–2
 Location, 28
 Locals, 29
 Prison, 32–3
 Prisoners, 32, 35–6
United States Army:
 555th Parachute Infantry Battalion, 149
 US Army Chemical Corps, 133, 135, 139
 US Coast Artillery, 45
United States Marine Corps:
 North China Marines, 51

Vasilevsky, Marshal Aleksandr, 123

Wainwright, Lt.-Gen. Jonathan, 65, 67, 72, 105
Waitt, Maj.-Gen. Alden, 139
Wakamatsu, Maj.-Gen. Yujiro, 34
Watkins, 1st Lt. Marvin, 106–107
Webb, Sir William, 138
Whelchel, Warren, 89–91, 98, 168–9
Wild, Maj. Cyril, 59–60
Williams, Lt.-Col. J.M., 52
Woosung Prison Camp (China), 51, 54, 69–70

Yamada, Gen. Otsuzo, 123, 141
Young, Sir Mark, 51, 69
Yuan Shi-kai, Gen., 14–15

Zhongma Fortress *see* Manchuria
Zhukov, Gen. Georgy, 15